MW01169105

INTERMITTENT FASTING FOR WOMEN OVER 50 REVOLUTION

A GUIDE TO HELP YOU LOSE WEIGHT WHILE GOING THROUGH MENOPAUSE, OPTIMIZE YOUR HEALTH, 28-DAY MEAL PLAN INCLUDED

EVA GREENWELL

CONTENTS

INTRODUCTION

Welcome, my dear reader. If you are here, it's because you've taken that courageous first step toward understanding and embracing a journey that is as transformational as it is personal: intermittent fasting, specially tailored for women over fifty. This space we're entering together is designed to be your sanctuary of empowerment, understanding, and unfailing support. Together, we will explore the nuances of a lifestyle that has the power to redefine our golden years.

My voyage into the world of intermittent fasting began amid the tumultuous waves of menopause. Like many women, I found myself grappling with unanticipated weight gain and bewildering shifts in my hormonal landscape. It was a period marked by frustration and a sense of loss—until I discovered the potent tool of intermittent fasting. This wasn't just another diet trend but a gateway to reclaiming my health, balance, and vitality. Along this journey, I encountered challenges, yes, but more importantly, I unearthed a wellspring of resilience and well-being that I'm eager to share with you.

What sets this book apart is its unwavering focus on you, the vibrant woman over fifty, navigating the complexities of menopausal changes. This isn't just about intermittent fasting. It's about crafting a holistic approach to health that marries the wisdom of nutrition, the balance of mental and emotional well-being, and the vitality of physical activity—all tailored uniquely to you. Here, we delve into customizable intermittent fasting plans, ensuring your path is effective and joyously sustainable.

As we unfold the pages together, you'll find that the book is segmented into digestible parts, each designed to guide you from understanding the foundational principles of intermittent fasting to integrating it seamlessly into your lifestyle. Expect to find practical advice grounded in the latest research and real stories of triumph from women like us. These narratives are not just stories but beacons of inspiration, illuminating our collective journey.

One of the most exhilarating aspects of this adventure is the concept of customizable intermittent fasting plans. Here, we recognize and celebrate that each of us is wonderfully unique. There's no one-size-fits-all approach; instead, you'll learn how to weave intermittent fasting into your life in a way that feels natural and fulfilling, aligned with your individual preferences, lifestyle, and health goals.

Along the way, we'll confront and dismantle the common myths and concerns surrounding intermittent fasting for our age group. Armed with evidence-based information, you'll be equipped to make informed decisions about your health, free from the shadows of doubt and misinformation.

And because no journey is complete without companions, this book includes an array of success stories from women over fifty who have transformed their lives through intermittent fasting.

Their diverse experiences serve not only as proof of what's possible but also as a mirror reflecting the myriad paths to success.

As you stand on the threshold of this empowering journey, consider yourself warmly invited to join a burgeoning community of like-minded women. Together, we are more than individuals seeking health; we are a movement redefining what it means to age with vitality and grace.

"Every new beginning comes from some other beginning's end." Let this be the end of wondering and the beginning of a journey filled with health, understanding, and joy. Welcome to the revolution.

CHAPTER 1

In the tapestry of life, the threads of health and well-being are interwoven with the delicate fibers of our biological essence. Within this intricate design, intermittent fasting emerges not merely as a method for managing weight but as a profound way to attune our bodies to their natural rhythms, enhancing overall vitality. This chapter unfurls the science behind intermittent fasting, shedding light on its profound impact on cellular and hormonal mechanisms. Here, we unravel the biological blueprint that underpins this practice, illustrating how it catalyzes a cascade of health-promoting processes.

INTERMITTENT FASTING: THE BIOLOGICAL BLUEPRINT

Understanding the Basics

At the heart of intermittent fasting lies a simple yet powerful principle: alternating cycles of eating and fasting. This pattern, echoing the eating habits of our ancestors, taps into the body's inherent mechanisms for adapting to periods without food. During fasting, the body shifts its energy sourcing, moving from glucose derived from food to ketones produced from stored fats. This transition is not just a mere change in fuel sources; it's a signal that initiates a series of beneficial cellular and hormonal responses. These responses are foundational to understanding the health benefits attributed to intermittent fasting.

Autophagy Activation

One of the most significant processes induced by intermittent fasting is autophagy, a term derived from the Greek words for "self" and "eating." This self-cleansing mechanism allows cells to degrade and recycle their components, removing damaged proteins and organelles. Think of autophagy as the body's internal maintenance system, cleansing cells of debris that, if accumulated, could lead to cellular dysfunction and disease. Activating autophagy through fasting is akin to hitting the reset button on our cells, promoting health and longevity. Studies, including those published in prestigious journals such as *Nature* and the *Journal of Clinical Investigation,* have highlighted autophagy's role in preventing diseases, including neurodegenerative disorders and cancer, by maintaining cellular integrity and function.

Insulin Sensitivity Improvement

Intermittent fasting's impact extends to metabolic health, mainly through its effect on insulin sensitivity. Insulin, a hormone produced by the pancreas, allows cells to absorb glucose from the bloodstream, using it for energy or storing it as fat. However, constant exposure to high levels of insulin, often a result of frequent eating, can lead to cells becoming less responsive to insulin signals, a condition known as insulin resistance. This resistance is a precursor to type 2 diabetes and a marker of metabolic syndrome. Intermittent fasting helps reverse this trend by reducing the demand for constant insulin production, allowing cells to regain their sensitivity to insulin. Enhanced insulin sensitivity supports healthy blood sugar levels and reduces the risk of metabolic diseases, marking a significant stride toward optimal health.

Impact on Growth Hormone

Another noteworthy benefit of intermittent fasting is its influence on growth hormone levels. Growth hormones play a pivotal role in health, regulating body composition by promoting muscle growth and fat breakdown. Its levels naturally decline with age, contributing to decreased muscle mass and increased fat that often accompanies aging. Fasting acts as a stimulant for growth hormone secretion. This increase not only aids in preserving muscle mass and encouraging fat use as an energy source but also supports the repair and regeneration of tissues throughout the body. The rise in growth hormone levels during fasting underscores the practice's utility in weight management and fostering overall muscular and metabolic health.

In weaving these threads together, the biological blueprint of intermittent fasting reveals a design intricately linked with our physiology. This alignment with our body's natural processes underscores the practice's efficacy, moving beyond diet trends to offer a foundation for lasting health and vitality. Through the lens of science, we see intermittent fasting not as a mere dietary intervention but as a return to a rhythm resonant with our biological heritage, promising a path to enhanced well-being.

Visual Element: The Cascade of Health Benefits

To visually encapsulate the cascade of benefits triggered by intermittent fasting, consider a flowchart diagram. This diagram begins with the initiation of intermittent fasting, branching into pathways representing autophagy activation, improved insulin sensitivity, and increased growth hormone levels. Each pathway culminates in the associated health benefits, such as enhanced cellular function, reduced risk of metabolic diseases, preservation of muscle mass, and efficient fat breakdown. This visual representation clarifies the interconnectedness of these processes and illustrates the comprehensive impact of intermittent fasting on health.

MENOPAUSE AND METABOLISM: NAVIGATING CHANGES

The onset of menopause signals a profound shift within the body. This metamorphosis extends beyond the cessation of fertility into the realm of metabolic reconfiguration. This period, often marked by fluctuations in weight and energy levels, beckons a closer examination of the underlying metabolic shifts. The crux of this transformation lies in the body's recalibration of energy expenditure and storage, a process subtly influenced by the waning of estrogen levels.

Metabolic Shifts

As women cross the threshold into menopause, they often encounter an unanticipated challenge: managing weight becomes markedly more difficult. This phenomenon is not a mere consequence of aging but a direct result of the body's metabolic adjustment to the changing hormonal landscape. The research elucidates that the metabolic rate—the engine governing calorie burn—

tapers off during menopause, leading to a propensity for weight accumulation and a noticeable dip in energy levels. The intricacies of this metabolic slowdown are not solely tied to hormonal changes but are compounded by a natural decline in muscle mass, further dampening the metabolic rate.

Estrogen's Role

Estrogen, once abundant, now dwindles, leaving a noticeable imprint on the body's metabolic machinery. This hormone, beyond its reproductive functions, plays a pivotal role in modulating metabolism, influencing how the body processes and stores fat. Its decline ushers in a tendency for fat to accumulate around the midsection, a pattern linked with heightened risks for cardiovascular disease and insulin resistance. Furthermore, estrogen's wane disrupts the delicate balance of leptin and ghrelin—hormones that regulate hunger and satiety—often leading to increased appetite and a consequent challenge in weight management.

Intermittent fasting emerges as a beacon of hope within this complex interplay of hormones and metabolism. By instigating periods of fasting, the body is coaxed into tapping into fat reserves for energy, circumventing the metabolic slowdown. More than a mere weight management tool, intermittent fasting rekindles the metabolic rate, offering a countermeasure to the energy lulls that often accompany menopause. It beckons a deeper understanding of how to align eating patterns with the body's evolved energy needs, crafting a harmonious existence with the metabolic shifts of menopause.

Adapting to Change

Adapting to the body's changing metabolic rate necessitates a thoughtful recalibration of diet and lifestyle. The cornerstone of this adaptation lies in synchronizing intermittent fasting schedules with the body's natural rhythms, fostering an environment where metabolism can thrive despite its slowed pace. This alignment not only aids in managing weight but also stabilizes energy levels, ensuring that fasting becomes a catalyst for vitality rather than a source of depletion. It prompts a reevaluation of physical activity, advocating for strength training to counteract muscle loss and further buoy the metabolic rate. This holistic approach, intertwining fasting with targeted exercise, paves a path through the metabolic maze of menopause, restoring balance and energy.

Thermogenic Foods

Within the dietary framework of intermittent fasting, including thermogenic foods offers a strategic advantage. These foods, known for their capacity to elevate the body's heat production, naturally enhance calorie burn, adding a layer of metabolic stimulation. Spices such as cayenne pepper and foods rich in omega-3 fatty acids, like salmon and green tea with their catechins, stand out for their thermogenic properties. Integrating these foods into the eating windows of an intermittent fasting regimen amplifies the metabolic rate. It enriches the diet with nutrients pivotal for menopausal health. This dietary strategy, woven into the fabric of intermittent fasting, acts as a lever, lifting the metabolic rate and aligning it with the body's adjusted energy dynamics.

In navigating the metabolic shifts of menopause, the confluence of intermittent fasting, strategic exercise, and the reasonable selection of foods becomes a tapestry of resilience. Within this tapestry, women find the strength to recalibrate their metabolism, embracing the changes wrought by menopause with informed grace and strategic action. The journey through menopause, with its myriad metabolic challenges, is not traversed by a singular path but through a mosaic of strategies, each tailored to the body's evolving needs. In this adaptation lies the power to redefine menopause, transforming it from a period of loss to one of renewal and vitality.

HORMONAL HARMONY: HOW FASTING AFFECTS ESTROGEN AND PROGESTERONE

In the intricate dance of a woman's body, hormones lead with a rhythm that dictates not just reproductive cycles but the overall symphony of health. Menopause introduces a shift in this rhythm, particularly in the levels of estrogen and progesterone, leading to a range of symptomatic expressions that can challenge well-being. In this context, intermittent fasting steps in, not as a mere dietary adjustment but as a conductor, aiming to restore harmony in the hormonal orchestra.

The balance between estrogen and progesterone is critical. Estrogen, known for its role in developing and maintaining female characteristics and reproductive systems, finds its counterpoint in progesterone, which is vital for regulating the menstrual cycle and supporting pregnancy. When these hormones become unbalanced, symptoms such as hot flashes, mood swings, and irregular periods can surface, signaling a disruption in the delicate equilibrium. Intermittent fasting, which influences insulin sensitivity and subsequently affects the hormonal milieu, can aid in moderating these fluctuations. It prompts a closer examination of adipose tissue's role as not just fat storage but as an endocrine organ itself, producing estrogen, which can contribute to the hormone imbalance experienced during menopause. By aiding in the reduction of fatty tissue, intermittent fasting can indirectly contribute to moderating estrogen levels, thus promoting a more balanced hormonal state.

Yet, the effectiveness of fasting on hormonal balance is not solely a matter of reducing adipose tissue. The timing of eating and fasting periods plays a crucial role in mitigating the hormonal swings that can exacerbate menopausal symptoms. Implementing a fasting schedule that aligns with natural circadian rhythms can help stabilize hormone levels throughout the day. For instance, it was concluded that the eating window should be early in the evening, thus aligning the fasting period with the body's natural inclination toward rest and repair during the night, which can support more stable levels of estrogen and progesterone. This alignment serves to smooth out the hormonal waves that can lead to the tumultuous symptoms associated with menopause.

Moreover, the symbiosis between intermittent fasting and exercise unveils another layer of hormonal regulation. Physical activity, especially strength training and aerobic exercises complements the hormonal balancing act of fasting. Exercise stimulates the release of endorphins, often called 'feel-good' hormones, which can alleviate stress and improve mood. Beyond the psychological benefits, exercise influences the body's sensitivity to insulin and, by extension, impacts the hormonal balance positively. When combined with intermittent fasting, exercise not only supports the maintenance of muscle mass—crucial for a healthy metabolic rate—but also promotes a more harmonious hormonal state, dampening the severity of menopausal symptoms.

Yet, not just the physical aspects of fasting and exercise merit attention, but also the psychological. Stress, an omnipresent factor in the modern landscape, profoundly impacts hormonal health, mainly through the secretion of cortisol, the stress hormone. High levels of cortisol can further unbalance estrogen and progesterone, adding to the complexity of managing menopausal symptoms. Mindful fasting practices emerge as a counterbalance to stress, encouraging a focus on the present and fostering a sense of control over one's health and body. Mindfulness during fasting can attenuate the stress response, moderating cortisol levels and, by extension, supporting a more balanced hormonal environment. Practices such as meditation, deep breathing, and even the mindful preparation and consumption of food during eating windows can transform the fasting experience into calm and reflection rather than stress and deprivation.

This nuanced approach to intermittent fasting, emphasizing timing, exercise, and mindfulness, transcends the traditional view of fasting as merely an interval between meals. It represents a holistic strategy for navigating the hormonal shifts of menopause, aiming not only to alleviate symptoms but to foster a state of well-being that resonates throughout the body's systems. Through this lens, intermittent fasting becomes more than a dietary pattern; it is a tool for reclaiming hormonal harmony and a sense of vitality and balance in the face of menopause challenges.

THE ROLE OF AUTOPHAGY IN AGING GRACEFULLY

In the orchestra of the body's mechanisms for maintenance and renewal, autophagy plays a first violin, its notes resonating with the promise of longevity and the diminution of the wear and tear accompanying aging. For women stepping into the post-menopausal phase of life, where cellular efficiency begins to wane, understanding and engaging in this process becomes pivotal. Autophagy, a term that means "self-eating," is the body's way of cleaning out damaged cells in order to regenerate newer, healthier cells. It's a recycling program at the cellular level, ensuring that the body's machinery runs smoothly by disposing of the old, damaged cellular components to make way for the new. This process is akin to an internal renovation, where the old and frail structures are demolished to make space for modern, efficient buildings that sustain the city's vigor and vitality.

Intermittent fasting acts as a catalyst for this cellular housekeeping. When the body is in a fasted state, the decrease in available glucose levels prompts cells to turn inward for energy, initiating the process of autophagy. It's as if the body, recognizing the absence of external nourishment, decides to conduct an internal audit, identifying and recycling components that no longer perform optimally. This provides an alternate energy source during fasting periods but also plays a critical role in preventing the accumulation of cellular debris. The importance of this process cannot be overstated, especially as one age, for it is the accumulation of damaged cellular components that is often at the heart of age-related decline.

The link between autophagy and disease prevention further underscores its significance. Age-related diseases, from neurodegeneration to cardiovascular issues, often find their roots in the failure of cellular components to maintain their integrity over time. Regularly inducing autophagy through intermittent fasting can proactively support the body's ability to fend off these diseases. It's a preventative measure to fortify the body's defenses by ensuring its cellular components remain as youthful and functional as possible. Research has illuminated the profound impact of autophagy on health, suggesting that enhanced autophagy can significantly extend lifespan and improve overall health. The connection between autophagy and reduced inflammation, a key contributor to many chronic diseases, further amplifies its role as a guardian of health in the later years of life.

Optimizing one's fasting schedule to maximize the benefits of autophagy requires a nuanced approach. It's not merely about the length of the fast but about finding a rhythm that aligns with one's unique physiological needs and lifestyle. While research suggests that autophagy ramps up after extended periods without food, typically beyond the 16-hour mark, plunging into prolonged fasts without preparation can lead to undue stress on the body. Instead, a gradual escalation allows the body to adapt, steadily increasing the fasting window while monitoring one's physical and mental response. This systematic approach ensures the fasting experience remains sustainable and beneficial, avoiding potential pitfalls such as nutritional deficiencies or undue fatigue.

In addition, syncing fasting periods with the body's circadian rhythm can enhance the effectiveness of autophagy. The body's biological clock governs myriad processes, including metabolism and cellular repair. By aligning fasting periods with this internal clock, one can potentiate the autophagic process, ensuring that cellular cleanup occurs in tandem with the body's natural tendencies toward repair during the nighttime. This synchronization between fasting and the circadian rhythm amplifies the restorative effects of sleep, turning each night into an opportunity for profound cellular rejuvenation.

Furthermore, the integration of nutrient-dense foods during eating windows plays a complementary role in supporting autophagy. Certain nutrients, such as polyphenols found in berries and green tea, as well as sulfur-rich vegetables like broccoli and onions, have been shown to encourage autophagy. Mindfully incorporating these foods into one's diet can bolster the autophagic process, ensuring that the body receives the raw materials necessary for optimal cellular renewal. This strategic approach to nutrition not only enhances the benefits of intermittent fasting but also ensures that the body remains nourished and resilient, capable of withstanding the rigors of fasting without compromise.

The dance between intermittent fasting, autophagy, and aging is a delicate one, requiring a thoughtful choreography that respects the body's limits while challenging its potential. In this intricate ballet, autophagy emerges as a key performer, its movements graceful yet potent, capable of transforming the landscape of aging into one of vitality and resilience. Through the lens of autophagy, intermittent fasting is revealed not just as a tool for weight management but as a profound ally in the quest for longevity, a beacon guiding women through the post-menopausal phase toward a horizon brimming with health and vitality.

DEBUNKING MYTHS: SEPARATING FACT FROM FICTION IN MENOPAUSAL HEALTH

In the realm of menopausal health and intermittent fasting, myths swirl like leaves in a storm, obscuring the path to understanding with their misleading dance. It's time to clear the air, to lay bare the truths hidden beneath layers of misconception, ensuring that clarity prevails over confusion.

The first myth that demands our attention is the oft-touted belief that intermittent fasting is unsuitable for menopausal women, that somehow, during this phase of life, the body becomes less capable of reaping the benefits of fasting. This notion stems from a misunderstanding of the body's resilience and adaptability. Far from being detrimental, intermittent fasting can be a linchpin in managing menopausal symptoms, enhancing metabolic health, and improving quality of life. Research, including studies published in journals such as *Aging* and *Cell Metabolism*, has consistently shown that intermittent fasting can lead to improvements in insulin sensitivity, reduction in inflammatory markers, and even enhancements in cognitive function—benefits that are particularly pertinent as we navigate the complexities of menopause.

Another pervasive myth is the idea that intermittent fasting leads to extreme hunger and discomfort, making it unsustainable in the long term. This belief underestimates the body's capability to adjust to new eating patterns. It overlooks the importance of a well-structured fasting plan. Hunger, while a natural initial response, diminishes over time as the body transitions to using stored fat for energy during fasting periods. Moreover, by focusing on nutrient-dense foods during eating windows and aligning fasting periods with the body's natural circadian rhythms, the sensation of hunger can be significantly mitigated, transforming the fasting experience from one of deprivation to one of rejuvenation.

In the face of these myths, the power of listening to one's body emerges as a guiding principle. The human body communicates its needs in a myriad of ways, from hunger pangs to the energy highs and lows that punctuate our days. Tuning into these signals allows us to navigate the fasting experience with sensitivity and awareness, adjusting our approach in response to our body's feedback. This attunement fosters a sense of harmony, ensuring that fasting supports rather than disrupts our well-being. It's a dialogue, a continuous exchange between our physiological needs and lifestyle choices, where attentiveness ensures that our fasting approach evolves in tandem with our body's changing needs.

Central to this dialogue is recognizing that customization is beneficial and imperative. The notion that a single fasting regimen could meet the needs of every woman navigating menopause is as reductive as it is unrealistic. Our bodies are as varied as our life stories, each with its own set of challenges, preferences, and goals. A fasting schedule that energizes one woman might leave another feeling drained; foods that nourish and satisfy one might not agree with another. This diversity demands a bespoke approach to intermittent fasting, one that considers the commonalities that unite us and the differences that make each of us unique.

Crafting a personalized fasting plan begins with exploring one's lifestyle, health goals, and nutritional needs. It takes into account not just the physiological aspects of fasting but also the practicalities of daily life. For some, a 16-hour fast may fit seamlessly into their routine, while for others, a more flexible approach, such as the 5:2 method, where two days a week are designated for reduced calorie intake, might be more manageable. The key lies in experimentation, approaching fasting with a spirit of curiosity and adaptability and being ready to adjust the plan in response to one's experiences and outcomes.

Beyond the structure of the fasting schedule, personalization extends to the composition of the diet. Here, the focus is on nutrient density to ensure that the foods consumed during eating windows provide a rich tapestry of vitamins, minerals, and other nutrients essential for health. This is particularly crucial during menopause, a time when the body's nutritional needs shift, requiring increased attention to bone health, cardiovascular health, and overall metabolic well-being. Incorporating a diverse array of whole foods, from leafy greens and colorful vegetables to lean proteins and healthy fats, ensures that the diet supports the body's needs, enhancing the efficacy of the fasting regimen.

In dispelling myths and embracing the principles of listening to one's body and customization, a path forward emerges. It's a path marked by clarity, grounded in evidence-based practices, and attuned to the unique needs of each individual. Here, intermittent fasting reveals its potential as a dietary pattern and a tool for empowerment—a means of navigating menopause with agency and intention. Through this lens, the journey through menopause becomes not a challenge to be endured but an opportunity for growth and discovery, a chance to redefine one's relationship with health and well-being.

UNDERSTANDING YOUR BODY'S SIGNALS: HUNGER, FULLNESS, AND HORMONAL CUES

In the realm of intermittent fasting, attuning oneself to the nuanced symphony of the body's signals becomes a vital skill. This attunement allows for a harmonious relationship between fasting and feeding, transforming what might initially appear as a rigorous regimen into a fluid and natural rhythm. Hunger and cravings, often mistaken as interchangeable, are, in fact, distinct cues that the body communicates, each bearing its own message and significance.

Hunger, a physiological necessity, signals the body's genuine need for nourishment. It emerges gradually, often accompanied by a sense of emptiness in the stomach and a decrease in energy levels, guiding us toward replenishment in a manner that respects our body's natural rhythms. Cravings, on the other hand, are more impulsive, a psychological urge driven by factors beyond the body's nutritional requirements. These can be triggered by emotional states, environmental cues, or even the mere sight or smell of food. This leads to a desire for specific tastes or textures that may not align with the body's actual needs.

Differentiating between these signals requires mindfulness, an intentional focus on the present moment that allows us to inter-pret our body's communications accurately. Mindful eating, a practice that encourages full attention to the experience of eating —savoring each bite, acknowledging the flavors, and noticing the effects on the body—serves as a bridge to understanding these signals. It fosters an awareness of fullness cues, those subtle shifts that signal satisfaction and contentment, averting the tendency to overeat during feeding windows. Moreover, mindfulness illuminates the hormonal cues that fluctuate throughout the menstrual cycle and menopause, affecting appetite and energy. By observing these patterns without judgment, one can adapt fasting and feeding practices to align with these hormonal shifts, ensuring that the approach to intermittent fasting remains responsive and supports the body's changing needs.

Adapting one's fasting plan based on this rich tapestry of bodily feedback is not a sign of inconsistency but a testament to the flexibility at the heart of a sustainable fasting practice. It acknowledges that the body is not a static entity but a dynamic system that responds to the ebb and flow of life's rhythms. Adjustments to the fasting schedule mean shortening or extending fasting periods based on energy levels, shifting eating windows to accommodate social engagements, or even allowing for a pause in fasting in response to heightened stress or illness. This adaptability ensures that intermittent fasting is not a rigid structure imposed upon life but a fluid practice that weaves seamlessly into the fabric of daily living.

Hydration plays a crucial role in this adaptability, serving both as a foundation for health and a tool for fine-tuning the fasting experience. The importance of hydration extends beyond the mere quenching of thirst; it is instrumental in managing hunger signals and enhancing satiety during fasting periods. Water, often overlooked in discussions of nutrition, can modulate the sensation of hunger, sometimes masking as hunger pangs when the body is actually in need of hydration. Ensuring adequate water intake, therefore, becomes a cornerstone of a well-managed fasting plan, helping to mitigate the intensity of hunger experienced during fasting windows and contributing to a sense of fullness during feeding times.

Moreover, hydration influences the body's metabolic processes, supporting the detoxification and cellular renewal activities that are amplified during fasting. It acts as a catalyst, facilitating the body's natural cleansing mechanisms and contributing to the overall effectiveness of the fasting regimen. Drinking water, infused with mindfulness, can become a ritual that anchors the fasting experience—a moment of pause and reflection amid the day's activities.

In this nuanced dance with the body's signals, intermittent fasting transforms from a mere dietary framework into a deep listening and responsiveness practice. It invites a dialogue with the body, a continuous exchange that deepens our understanding of our needs and rhythms. Through this dialogue, fasting becomes not an imposition but an expression of self-care, a testament to the body's resilience and our capacity for attunement.

In navigating the signals of hunger, fullness, and hormonal cues, we find a space for growth and adaptation, a terrain where the practice of intermittent fasting evolves in harmony with our body's wisdom. This evolution reflects a commitment not to a rigid regimen but to a sustainable practice that honors the body's signals and supports its journey toward health and vitality. It is in this commitment that the true essence of intermittent fasting is revealed, not as a path marked by deprivation but as a journey enriched by awareness, flexibility, and a deepened connection with oneself.

CUSTOMIZING YOUR INTERMITTENT FASTING EXPERIENCE

The canvas of our lives is painted with the daily routines, the ebb and flow of social engagements, and the unique tapestry of our personal and family commitments. Within this intricate design, finding the perfect fasting window is akin to discovering the golden hour for a photographer—that pristine moment where everything aligns, and the result is nothing short of magical. This chapter guides you through evaluating your lifestyle to seamlessly integrate intermittent fasting, ensuring it complements rather than complicates your life.

ASSESSING YOUR LIFESTYLE FOR THE PERFECT FASTING WINDOW

Lifestyle Evaluation

Imagine planning a garden; you wouldn't plant shade-loving ferns in the sun's full glare. Similarly, selecting a fasting window requires understanding the terrain of your daily life. Reflect on your routine, sleep patterns, and physical activity levels. For someone who revels in morning hush, savoring breakfast as a ritualistic start to the day, an eating window that omits morning nourishment might cast a shadow over their dawn. Conversely, night owls, thriving in the late hours, might find an early eating window that truncates their vibrant evenings.

Fasting Types Overview

Intermittent fasting comes in varied landscapes: the 16/8 method, where you fast for 16 hours and eat during an 8-hour window, suits those who find simplicity in skipping breakfast. The 5:2 approach—eating normally for five days and reducing calorie intake for two—offers flexibility for those with fluctuating schedules. OMAD (One Meal a Day) draws a picture of simplicity yet requires resilience of spirit and a well-thought-out plan to meet nutritional needs in a single sitting. Each method has its rhythm; finding harmony within these can transform your experience from enduring to thriving.

Trial and Error

In the spirit of a scientist, approach this phase with curiosity. If the 16/8 method leaves you feeling drained by mid-afternoon, consider adjusting your eating window or experimenting with the 5:2 method. It's not about steadfastly adhering to a chosen method but about listening and adapting, finding what truly resonates with your body's needs and your lifestyle's demands.

Social and Family Considerations

Dinner with family isn't just about the food on the table; it's a tapestry of interaction, shared stories, and laughter. Integrating fasting into your life shouldn't mean isolating yourself from these moments. If family dinners are the cornerstone of your day, plan your eating window to ensure you're part of this communal joy. It's about weaving fasting into the fabric of your life, not unraveling the threads that hold it together.

Textual Element: Integrating Intermittent Fasting into Your Life

A checklist serves as a tangible tool to navigate the integration of intermittent fasting into your daily life:

- Daily Routine Check: Mark out when you're most energetic and feel sluggish. Align your eating window to support your energy peaks.
- Social Calendar Sync: Look ahead at your social commitments. Plan fasting windows that allow participation without compromise.
- Family Meal Mapping: Identify the main meals shared with the family and ensure your eating window captures these moments.
- Activity Adjustment: Note the times you're most physically active. Align your nutrient intake to support these periods of heightened activity.

Finding the perfect fasting window is an art and science in the confluence of daily demands and personal health goals. It requires a keen understanding of one's rhythms and routines, a willingness to adapt, and a commitment to integrate fasting seamlessly into the tapestry of life. Through careful consideration and thoughtful adjustment, intermittent fasting becomes not just a method for health optimization but a harmonious element of your daily existence.

TYPES OF FASTING PLANS: WHICH ONE IS RIGHT FOR YOU?

In the realm of intermittent fasting, a variety of strategies unfold, each with its own rhythm and requirements. This diversity ensures that anyone, regardless of their daily patterns or health aspirations, can find a method that resonates with their lifestyle. However, choosing the most suitable plan demands a deep dive into the specifics of each approach, considering not only the logistical aspects but also how they align with individual health goals and pre-existing medical conditions.

Detailed Plan Descriptions

The landscape of intermittent fasting is rich and varied, encompassing methods like the Eat-Stop-Eat, where 24-hour fasts are undertaken once or twice a week, offering a reset for the digestive system and a profound sense of accomplishment upon completion. Another approach, the Warrior Diet, advocates for a 20-hour fasting window followed by a 4-hour eating window, ideally filled with nutrient-dense foods, catering to those who find liberation in minimal daytime eating and a hearty evening meal. Meanwhile, Alternate Day Fasting presents a rhythm of day-on, day-off eating, which, though demanding, provides flexibility and significant metabolic benefits. Each method carries its advantages and challenges—from the simplicity of adherence to the intensity of the fasting periods—necessitating a thoughtful evaluation of how each aligns with personal health objectives and daily routines.

The 24-Hour Fast: Incorporating Monthly Resets

In the journey toward a healthier lifestyle, intermittent fasting has emerged as a transformative approach, particularly beneficial for women over fifty. The 24-hour fast stands out for its simplicity and profound health benefits among various fasting methods. This chapter delves into the purpose of 24-hour fasts, offering guidance on planning, execution, and optimal frequency to harness its benefits while ensuring it complements your lifestyle and health needs.

Purpose of 24-Hour Fasts

A 24-hour fast, also known as a full-day fast, involves abstaining from food for a full day. It's a powerful tool to reset your body and mind, providing numerous health benefits:

- Detoxification: Fasting initiates autophagy, a cellular "cleanup" process that removes damaged cells and generates new ones. This process is crucial for detoxifying the body and promoting longevity.
- Mental Clarity: Many fasters report enhanced mental clarity and focus during and after a 24-hour fast. This mental boost is attributed to reduced blood sugar fluctuations and increased brain-derived neurotrophic factor (BDNF) production.
- Insulin Sensitivity Improvement: Regularly practicing 24-hour fasts can help improve insulin sensitivity, reduce the risk of type 2 diabetes, and support weight management.
- Inflammation Reduction: Fasting has been shown to decrease markers of inflammation, a key factor in chronic diseases.

Planning Your Fast

Successfully incorporating a 24-hour fast into your routine requires preparation, mindful execution, and a proper strategy to break the fast. Here's how to plan for success:

- Preparation: In the days before your fast, focus on hydrating well and eating nutrient-dense foods. This preparation helps ease the transition into fasting and supports your body throughout the process.
- Execution: During the fast, stay hydrated with water, herbal teas, or black coffee. Keep yourself occupied with light activities such as walking, reading, or meditative practices. Listen to your body, and if you feel unwell, consider adjusting the duration of the fast.
- Breaking the Fast: Break your fast gently with a light meal rich in vegetables, lean proteins, and healthy fats. Avoid heavy, processed, or sugary foods that can shock your digestive system.

Frequency Recommendations

The frequency of 24-hour fasts can vary depending on individual health goals, lifestyle, and how your body responds to fasting. For women over fifty, incorporating a 24-hour fast once a month is a good starting point. This frequency supports detoxification and health benefits without imposing undue stress on the body.

As you become more accustomed to fasting, consider adjusting the frequency, possibly increasing it to twice a month. However, the focus should always be on quality and sustainability over quantity.

Listening to Your Body

A central tenet of successful intermittent fasting, especially for women over fifty, is tuning into your body's signals. During a 24-hour fast, it's crucial to be mindful of how you feel and make adjustments as necessary. Suppose you experience intense discomfort, weakness, or other adverse symptoms. In that case, it's essential to consider ending the fast early or consulting with a healthcare professional.

Personal Goals and Preferences

Aligning a fasting plan with personal health goals and preferences is akin to selecting the right gear for a long-awaited expedition; the compatibility between the two can significantly impact the journey's success. For individuals targeting weight loss, methods with extended fasting periods, such as alternate-day Day Fasting, might offer accelerated results. In contrast, those seeking improved metabolic health might find the consistent daily rhythm of the 16/8 method more conducive to sustaining long-term changes. This alignment extends beyond health objectives to encompass lifestyle preferences, where the feasibility of a fasting plan is intricately linked to one's daily commitments and social life. For instance, the flexibility of the 5:2 method might appeal to those with fluctuating schedules, enabling them to adapt fasting days to their social and work calendars.

Medical Conditions and Fasting

Navigating the intersection of intermittent fasting and existing medical conditions requires a nuanced understanding of how fasting impacts various health issues. Conditions such as diabetes or hypoglycemia necessitate careful monitoring and possibly adaptations to fasting plans to ensure blood sugar levels remain stable. Similarly, individuals with thyroid disorders must consider how fasting might affect thyroid hormone production and metabolism. This consideration underscores the importance of consulting healthcare professionals when choosing a fasting method, ensuring it supports overall health without exacerbating pre-existing conditions. It is not merely about pursuing health goals but about fostering well-being that acknowledges and respects the body's medical landscape.

Success Stories

The narratives of women who have successfully woven intermittent fasting into the fabric of their lives illuminate the potential of this lifestyle to transform health and well-being. For instance, a woman in her late fifties shares how the 16/8 method facilitated weight loss and instilled a sense of discipline and empowerment in her dietary choices, sustaining her energy levels and metabolic health. Another recounts her journey with the Warrior Diet, finding an unexpected liberation from food-related anxiety in its stringent fasting window, alongside noticeable improvements in digestive health. These stories, diverse in their outcomes and methods, serve as testaments to the adaptability of intermittent fasting, offering insights and motivation to those at the threshold of their fasting journey. They underscore that success in intermittent fasting is not measured solely by achieving specific health metrics but by cultivating a harmonious lifestyle with one's personal health aspirations and daily realities.

In this exploration of fasting plans, the emphasis lies not only on the logistical details of each method but also on the alignment between these strategies and the intricate mosaic of individual lives. It is a process that marries the practical with the personal, ensuring that the chosen path of intermittent fasting resonates deeply, supports health, and enhances the quality of life. This alignment, carefully crafted and continuously tuned, paves the way for a fasting experience that is not only sustainable but profoundly transformative.

ADJUSTING YOUR FASTING PLAN AS YOUR BODY ADAPTS

In intermittent fasting, listening to one's body is not merely a suggestion but a necessity. Much like a gardener attentively read the signs of the soil and plants to provide the proper care, you, too, must become attuned to the subtle and not-so-subtle signals your body sends. This attunement is crucial as your body undergoes the numerous changes that fasting instigates, requiring a readiness to adapt your fasting plan in response to these evolving needs.

Listening and Adapting

The principle of adaptation lies at the heart of any successful intermittent fasting strategy. It recognizes the dynamic nature of the human body—a living system in constant flux, responding to internal and external stimuli. As such, a fasting regimen that once seemed to fit perfectly with your lifestyle and health goals may, over time, require adjustments. This realization is not an indication of failure but a testament to your body's ongoing adaptation process. Listening—truly listening to your body—involves an openness to recognize when changes are necessary and the courage to implement them. It's about observing not just the evident shifts in weight or energy levels but also the subtler cues, such as changes in mood, sleep quality, and digestion, which can all signal the need for a new approach.

Sigs for Adjustment

Recognizing the need for adjustment in your fasting plan often begins with an awareness of your body's rhythms and responses. Signs that indicate a need for change include persistent energy dips, sleep disturbances, or a plateau in weight loss goals. Energy dips, for example, could manifest as a lethargic drag in the afternoons, a time when you previously felt vibrant and alert. Sleep disturbances arise not just as difficulty in falling asleep but as changes in sleep quality, perhaps waking frequently throughout the night or experiencing restless sleep. These signals serve as your body's communication, a nudge to reevaluate and adjust your fasting schedule or approach to better align with your current state of health and well-being.

Gradual Changes

When the time comes to adjust your fasting plan, adopting a strategy of gradual change is pivotal. Sudden, sweeping modifications can shock the system, leading to discomfort or a sense of overwhelm that may deter you from continuing. Instead, consider minor, incremental adjustments akin to softly turning the dial to fine-tune the radio reception. If extending your fasting window, do so in small increments, perhaps by 30 minutes to an hour, allowing your body to acclimate to the new rhythm. Similarly, if adjusting your eating window to earlier in the day to combat energy slumps, shift gradually to help your body and mind adapt without resistance. This approach ensures that changes are sustainable in the long term, woven into the fabric of your lifestyle with care and consideration.

Seeking Professional Guidance

Professional guidance becomes invaluable in personalizing and adjusting your intermittent fasting plan at certain junctures. This need might arise from specific health concerns, such as managing chronic conditions or navigating complex nutritional needs, where the insight of a healthcare provider or a registered dietitian can illuminate the path forward. Seeking professional guidance is a step imbued with the recognition that, while much can be achieved through self-directed learning and experimentation, the complexities of health and nutrition often require a deeper, more nuanced understanding. It's about partnering with professionals who can offer tailored advice grounded in scientific knowledge and clinical experience to refine your fasting plan in ways that support your health holistically.

In this adaptation journey, where listening to your body is as critical as fasting, remember that change is inevitable and necessary. Through this lens of adaptability, gradual change, and, when needed, professional insight, intermittent fasting transcends the realm of diet and emerges as a sustainable practice. This practice honors the body's ever-changing needs on the path to health and vitality.

COMBINING INTERMITTENT FASTING WITH YOUR CURRENT DIET

In the nuanced ballet of nutrition and health, marrying intermittent fasting with an existing diet mirrors the intricate pairing of fine wine with a gourmet meal, where each component enhances the other, creating a symphony of flavors and benefits. This harmonization demands a deep understanding of the distinct rhythms of fasting and various dietary frameworks and an appreciation for the unique nutritional tapestry of each individual, especially women navigating the complexities of life beyond fifty.

Integration with Dietary Preferences

The fusion of intermittent fasting with dietary preferences such as vegan, ketogenic, or Mediterranean diets emerges as a dance of balance and harmony. For the vegan adherent, this integration involves a meticulous orchestration of plant-based proteins, fats, and carbohydrates within the eating windows, ensuring a rich tapestry of nutrients that supports both the fasting journey and the ethical commitment to veganism. On the other hand, the ketogenic enthusiast finds a potent amplification of metabolic flexibility in this combination, as the body, already primed to tap into fat for fuel, navigates the fasting periods with heightened efficiency and ease. Meanwhile, with its cornucopia of whole grains, lean proteins, and heart-healthy fats, the Mediterranean diet offers a lush backdrop for intermittent fasting, ensuring that each meal celebrates taste and health.

Nutritional Considerations

Ensuring nutritional balance and adequacy becomes paramount in this confluence of dietary practices, particularly for women over fifty, who stand at the threshold of increased nutritional needs and metabolic shifts. The challenge here is not merely in avoiding caloric excess or deficiency but in the meticulous weaving of a nutritional quilt that blankets the body with a spectrum of vitamins, minerals, and other phytonutrients essential for thriving health. This endeavor requires a vigilant eye for detail—calcium and vitamin D for bone health, iron to fend off anemia, and omega-3 fatty acids for cognitive and cardiovascular well-being. Each nutrient and vitamin becomes a thread in the fabric of health, woven with intention and care into the eating windows of intermittent fasting.

Flexibility and Forgiveness

Amid the rigor of combining diets, the principles of flexibility and forgiveness stand as beacons of grace, illuminating the path with understanding and self-compassion. This journey is not one of rigid adherence but of fluid exploration, where deviations are not failures but opportunities for learning and growth. The missed fasting window and unintended indulgence are not defeats but reminders of our humanity, moments to practice forgiveness and recommit to our health goals with renewed vigor. In this space, flexibility becomes our ally, allowing us to easily navigate social engagements and unexpected life events, ensuring that our dietary practices enhance rather than constrict our lives.

Case Studies

In the tapestry of real-world experiences, stories of women who have seamlessly blended intermittent fasting with their dietary preferences emerge as vibrant threads, each narrating a tale of adaptation, challenge, and triumph. Consider the story of a woman in her late fifties, a devout follower of the Mediterranean diet, who discovered a renewed sense of vitality in intermittent fasting and a significant reduction in inflammatory markers. Her journey, marked by a careful selection of nutrient-dense foods within her eating windows, illustrates this dietary fusion's potential to support weight management and foster a deeper connection with food as a source of nourishment and joy.

Another narrative unfolds with a woman who embraced the ketogenic diet in her quest for metabolic health, finding intermittent fasting an unexpected ally. The synergy between her high-fat, low-carbohydrate diet and the fasting periods propelled her into a state of sustained ketosis, enhancing her mental clarity and energy levels and offering a testament to the power of dietary integration to transform health.

These stories, each unique in their contours and outcomes, serve as testimonials to intermittent fasting's adaptability and capacity to meld with various dietary frameworks in a way that supports individual health goals, preferences, and lifestyles. They stand as proof of concept, not just for the feasibility of combining diets but also for the profound impact such a combination can have on overall well-being.

In this exploration of combining intermittent fasting with existing dietary preferences, the emphasis shifts from the prescriptive to the personal, from a one-size-fits-all approach to a bespoke journey tailored to the individual. It is a journey marked by balance, nutritional attentiveness, and an open heart, where flexibility and forgiveness pave the way for a harmonious integration of fasting and dietary practices. This fusion, carefully nurtured and attentively adjusted, promises enhanced physical health and a deeper, more fulfilling relationship with food and nutrition.

THE IMPORTANCE OF HYDRATION AND SUPPLEMENTS

In the tapestry of well-being that women over fifty weaves through intermittent fasting, threads of hydration and supplements intertwine to form a crucial support structure. This framework enhances the efficacy of fasting and ensures that the body's intricate system maintains its equilibrium, particularly during the ebb of the fasting phase.

Hydration's Critical Role

The significance of hydration transcends the simplicity of quenching thirst; it is the lifeblood of cellular function and a cornerstone of health, especially during fasting. Water is a medium for transporting nutrients, a catalyst for biochemical reactions, and a lubricant for joints and tissues. During fasting periods, the absence of food intake means the body misses out on the additional water sourced from fruits, vegetables, and other foods, making deliberate water consumption even more vital. The aim is to maintain an optimal level of hydration that supports the body's metabolic processes, aids in eliminating toxins, and ensures the smooth operation of bodily functions. Emphasizing water intake, herbal teas, and electrolyte-infused beverages can mitigate common fasting side effects such as headaches and fatigue, directly impacting one's ability to sustain fasting over the long term.

Supplement Recommendations

Navigating the landscape of supplements during intermittent fasting requires a discerning eye, particularly for women over fifty whose nutritional needs are distinct. The objective is to fill any dietary gaps that must be fully addressed through diet alone, especially considering the condensed eating windows. Vitamins D and B12, often challenging to obtain in adequate amounts from food, stand out as pivotal for bone health and energy metabolism. Magnesium and calcium are vital for muscle function and bone density, and their importance is magnified in the post-menopausal years. Omega-3 fatty acids, sourced from fish oil or algae supplements, contribute to cardiovascular health and cognitive function, offering a buffer against the decline often associated with aging. In selecting supplements, the focus should remain on quality and bioavailability, ensuring that the body can efficiently utilize these nutrients to support health and vitality during fasting.

Electrolyte Balance

The tapestry of health is delicately balanced on the fulcrum of electrolytes—minerals such as sodium, potassium, magnesium, and calcium, pivotal in regulating hydration, nerve signals, and muscle function. During fasting, the body's electrolyte balance can shift, particularly with the loss of sodium and potassium through reduced food intake and increased water consumption. Maintaining this balance is not merely about preventing dehydration but sustaining the electrical gradients that drive nerve transmission and muscle contraction, essential for every heartbeat and thought. Incorporating electrolyte-rich beverages or supplements can help maintain this balance, ensuring that fasting does not disrupt the body's symphony of electrical activity. Mindful of the quantities and sources, women can navigate fasting without compromising this delicate equilibrium.

Consulting Healthcare Providers

The decision to integrate supplements into a fasting regimen is neither taken lightly nor in isolation. Engaging with healthcare providers offers an indispensable layer of insight, tailoring supplement choices to individual health profiles and needs. This dialogue is particularly pertinent for women over fifty, where considerations such as medication interactions, pre-existing conditions, and specific nutritional deficiencies come into play. Healthcare providers can offer guidance on appropriate supplement types, dosages, and timing, ensuring that supplementation complements rather than complicates the fasting experience. This partnership, grounded in professional expertise and personal health history, ensures that the hydration and supplementation approach is safe and effective, supporting women in their fasting endeavors without detracting from their overall health objectives.

In weaving hydration and supplements into the fabric of intermittent fasting, the aim is to support the physical body and enhance the overall fasting experience, making it a sustainable and enriching practice. It is about creating a foundation that bolsters the body's resilience, ensuring that women over fifty can navigate the ebb and flow of fasting with grace and vitality. This framework, carefully constructed and attentively maintained, becomes an integral part of the fasting journey, a testament to the power of informed and mindful practice in achieving health and well-being.

SETTING REALISTIC GOALS AND TRACKING PROGRESS

Setting goals is a balanced practice in the nuanced realm of personal health and wellness, particularly for women navigating the transformative period of their fifties and beyond. It is the delicate act of aiming for the stars while keeping one's feet firmly planted on the ground. Realistic, achievable goals serve not only as beacons of motivation but as tangible milestones that map the path to success in intermittent fasting. Therefore, crafting these goals demands not just ambition but a profound understanding of one's capacities, limitations, and the intricate dance of life's responsibilities.

Crafting such goals begins with a reflective and informed reflection, considering not just the desired outcomes but the journey required to attain them. It's about envisioning success not as a distant peak but as a series of attainable ledges, each offering a vantage point to appreciate progress. Whether it's aiming to integrate fasting into one's lifestyle without disrupting family meals or enhancing energy levels to support a newfound hobby, the specificity of these goals lends them their power. They become aspirations and actionable objectives, each tailored to fit the unique contours of one's life.

With goals set, the journey then transitions to tracking progress, a practice that is as varied as it is vital. In this digital age, apps offer a convenient and comprehensive means to monitor fasting schedules, nutritional intake, and physical activity, allowing for a holistic view of one's progress. Yet, for those who find solace in the tactile, journals provide a canvas not just for logging meals and fasting windows but for reflecting on the emotional and psychological facets of the fasting experience. Body measurements, too, offer a tangible metric of change, capturing the physical transformations that accompany dedication and discipline. Yet, these methods are but tools, each selected and utilized based on personal preference and the specific nuances of one's goals.

Beyond the scale, non-scale victories emerge as a vital component of tracking progress. These victories, often overlooked, are the subtle yet significant signs of improvement that transcend numerical metrics. An increased vitality that imbues one's mornings with zest, a serenity in sleep that was once elusive, or a buoyancy in mood that colors one's interactions are the markers of success that often matter most. Celebrating these victories is not just an act of recognition but a reinforcement of the positive changes that intermittent fasting brings into one's life, serving as a wellspring of motivation as one navigates the highs and lows of the fasting journey.

Yet, the path is not static, and as one progresses, the necessity of adjusting goals becomes apparent. This adjustment is not an admission of miscalculation but an acknowledgment of growth, an understanding that as one evolves, so, too, do one's needs, preferences, and capacities. This fluidity in goal setting ensures that objectives remain relevant and aligned with one's current state, encouraging a perpetual forward momentum that is both adaptive and reflective of personal development. It is a reminder that goals are not fixed stars in the sky but lanterns on a path that winds and shifts, illuminating the way forward.

In the intricate weave of setting realistic goals, tracking progress, celebrating non-scale victories, and adjusting objectives, the narrative of intermittent fasting unfolds not as a rigid regimen but as a dynamic, evolving practice. It is a practice rooted in self-awareness, nurtured by diligence, and enriched by celebrating the grand and granular improvements in one's health and well-being. This approach, grounded in realism and buoyed by optimism, offers a blueprint for success in intermittent fasting and a philosophy for approaching life's broader challenges with grace and grit.

As this chapter closes, it leaves behind the essence of a journey marked by intention, reflection, and adaptability. It paints a picture of a path walked with purpose, where goals are set with wisdom, progress is monitored with an eye for the holistic, and adjustments are made with the fluidity of a river carving its course through the landscape. This narrative, rich with the lessons of perseverance and the joys of discovery, lays the groundwork for the following exploration, inviting a deeper dive into the nourishing world of meal planning and the culinary delights in the next chapter.

MASTERING NUTRITION DURING YOUR EATING WINDOWS

In the quiet moments before dawn breaks, there's a world awakening within the kitchen. It's where the day's first decisions are made, not with a grand plan but with the simple act of choosing what to eat. This seemingly small choice ripples outward, influencing energy levels, mood, and overall well-being. For women over fifty, these choices carry even more weight as the body's needs evolve, making the dance between fasting and feeding not just a routine but a vital part of maintaining health and vitality. Here, the focus turns to the building blocks of life itself: macro- and micronutrients. These are the threads from which the fabric of health is woven; each meal is an opportunity to strengthen this intricate tapestry.

MACRO AND MICRONUTRIENTS: BUILDING A BALANCED DIET

Understanding Nutrient Categories

At the heart of nutrition lies a distinction crucial for understanding how to nourish the body effectively: macronutrients and micronutrients. The former, comprising carbohydrates, proteins, and fats, are the fuels that power the body's daily operations. They're the dense forests from which the body harvests energy, with each tree—whether a towering carbohydrate, a sturdy protein, or a resilient fat—playing a unique role in the body's ecosystem. Micronutrients, though smaller in stature, are no less vital. These vitamins and minerals, scattered like seeds throughout the diet, are essential for the body's processes, from bone health to energy production.

Balancing Act

Creating a balanced diet is akin to composing a symphony, with each nutrient a note that must harmonize with the others to produce a masterpiece. For women over fifty, this balance is delicate; the body's needs are nuanced. Carbohydrates, often vilified, are the body's preferred source of energy, especially important for fueling brain function. Yet, choosing carbohydrates matters profoundly, with whole grains, fruits, and vegetables providing the slow-burning energy sustained through fasting periods. Proteins, the building blocks of muscle and tissue, become crucial as the body loses muscle mass with age. Fats, mainly those rich in omega-3 fatty acids, support brain health and reduce inflammation. Achieving this balance means meeting the body's energy needs and supporting its overall function and health.

Nutrient-Dense Foods

In the garden of nutrition, some plants are more nourishing than others. Nutrient-dense foods packed with vitamins and minerals are the powerhouses of the diet. Dark, leafy greens, vibrant berries, lean proteins, and nuts and seeds are just a few examples. Incorporating these into the eating window doesn't just fill the stomach; it enriches the body's stores of essential nutrients, supporting everything from immune function to heart health. These foods are necessary for women over fifty, offering a concentrated source of nutrients to support health through menopause and beyond.

Supplementation Considerations

Even the most carefully tended gardens have gaps where the soil needs more nutrients for the plants to thrive. In the diet, these gaps are often filled with supplements, especially for micronutrients that are hard to obtain in sufficient quantities through food alone. Vitamin D usually called the "sunshine vitamin," is a nutrient crucial for bone health but challenging to get from diet alone. Iron, vital for carrying oxygen through the blood, and B12, essential for nerve function and energy production, are others. For women over fifty, a thoughtful approach to supplementation can ensure that the body receives all it needs to thrive, even within the constraints of an intermittent fasting schedule.

Textual Element: Your Nutritional Toolkit

A checklist serves as a practical guide for weaving macro- and micronutrients into the fabric of your diet:

- Daily Macros Check: Ensure each meal contains a balance of carbohydrates, proteins, and fats tailored to your body's needs and activity levels.
- Micronutrient Magnifying Glass: Focus on foods rich in vitamins and minerals crucial for women over fifty, such as calcium, vitamin D, and iron.
- Powerhouse Foods: Incorporate at least one serving of nutrient-dense foods into each meal, aiming for various colors and types.
- Supplement Strategy: Identify potential nutritional gaps and consult a healthcare provider about appropriate supplements to fill these needs.

In the quiet of the morning kitchen, as choices unfold with the breaking dawn, selecting what to eat becomes an act of self-care, a moment to nourish not just the body but the soul. For women over fifty, these choices are guided by understanding macros and micros, a balance between energy and enrichment, and the wisdom to supplement when necessary. This is where health begins, not with grand gestures but with the simple, everyday act of eating.

ANTI-INFLAMMATORY FOODS FOR MENOPAUSAL WOMEN

In the quiet revolution within, where the body seeks equilibrium amid the whispers of menopause and the advancing years, inflammation emerges as an uninvited guest, unsettling this balance.

Often unnoticed, this subtle yet persistent inflammation lays the groundwork for discomfort and various age-related ailments. It is here, in this delicate arena, that the inclusion of anti-inflammatory foods becomes not just a choice but a necessity, a means to soothe and quiet the internal tumult that accompanies the transition through menopause and beyond.

The arsenal against inflammation is vast, stocked with foods and spices that carry the dual mantle of flavor and healer. Omega-3-rich salmon and flaxseeds are among the vanguard, renowned for their ability to quell inflammation's flames. Their companions, the vibrant berries and the verdant kale, come laden with antioxidants, each a warrior against oxidative stress that fuels inflammation's fire. Together, these foods form a coalition, a united front in the body's ongoing struggle against the creeping tide of inflammation that seeks to undermine health and vitality.

Yet, it is not only in the fruits of the sea and the fields that relief is found but also in the bounty of the spice rack. Turmeric, with its golden hue and centuries-old lineage as a medicinal root, stands out for its curcumin content, a compound lauded for its anti-inflammatory prowess. With its sharp bite, ginger follows closely, offering a kick to dishes and a blow to inflammation. These spices, along with their brethren—garlic with its sulfurous compounds, cinnamon with its sweet warmth, and rosemary with its aromatic oils—transform meals from mere sustenance into potent elixirs of health.

Crafting a diet that weaves these anti-inflammatory staples into the fabric of daily eating requires knowledge and creativity. It invites a reimagining of meals, where salmon becomes the star of the dinner plate, flanked by a kale salad sprinkled with flaxseeds and berries. It sees soups and stews infused with ginger and turmeric, their colors deepening as the spices release their healing properties into the broth. This culinary creativity extends to snacks, where nuts and seeds, each a mini trove of anti-inflammatory power, become the go-to for midday hunger, replacing the processed, sugar-laden foods that often exacerbate inflammation.

The personalization of this anti-inflammatory crusade is crucial, recognizing that the map to well-being is not universal but deeply individual. It acknowledges the unique tapestry of preferences, intolerances, and dietary restrictions that each woman brings to the table. For some, the path may be laden with grains and legumes. Still, their vegetarian heart finds solace and sustenance in the plant kingdom. For others, the journey may weave through the waters, pescatarian choices offering a compromise between the land and the sea. And yet, for others, the exploration may embrace the vast expanse of the dietary spectrum, finding balance and health in the moderation of all things.

This journey is guided not by stringent rules but by gentle principles, a framework within which creativity and personal taste are not just allowed but encouraged. It is supported by resources—a curated list of anti-inflammatory foods, a collection of recipes that inspire and nourish, and a network of communities that share in the quest for health through the healing power of food. These resources, readily available and endlessly adaptable, offer not just guidance but inspiration, fueling the transformation of the diet from a source of potential inflammation to a wellspring of healing.

In this endeavor, the role of the kitchen transforms, becoming not just a place of meal preparation but a sanctuary of health creation. Here, the battle against inflammation is fought not with drugs and interventions but with chopping boards and spices, with the sizzle of olive oil in the pan and the vibrant hues of vegetables on the plate. This culinary alchemy, where ingredients are transformed into healing meals, becomes a daily ritual, a practice of self-care that extends its benefits far beyond the confines of the kitchen.

In the end, the incorporation of anti-inflammatory foods into the diet emerges as a testament to the power of nutrition, a reminder that within the realm of food lies the potential for disease and the promise of health and vitality. It is a choice, made daily, to nourish the body with what it needs to heal, to thrive, and to navigate the transitions of life with strength and grace.

BONE HEALTH: CALCIUM, VITAMIN D, AND BEYOND

In the quiet theater of the body's inner workings, a complex interplay unfolds daily, a silent ballet where calcium, vitamin D, and other nutrients perform in a delicate balance to maintain bone strength and density. This equilibrium becomes particularly poignant for women over fifty as the curtain rises on a stage where the risk of osteoporosis looms large, casting long shadows over the future of their mobility and independence. Herein lies not just a tale of sustenance but one of strategic nourishment, where every meal becomes an opportunity to fortify the skeletal framework that supports not merely the body but the very essence of vitality.

Calcium is the cornerstone of this skeletal fortification, a mineral renowned for creating the bone matrix and sustaining its density. Yet, its efficacy is intricately tied to vitamin D, a luminary that facilitates calcium's absorption and utilization within the body. This partnership is critical; a harmonious alliance ensures calcium's journey from the digestive tract to the bone tissue is efficient and effective. However, the narrative of bone health extends beyond these two protagonists to include the supporting cast of vitamin K, magnesium, and phosphorus, each contributing to the intricate bone renewal and repair process. Vitamin K, particularly in its K2 form, directs calcium to the bones, deterring it from depositing in the arteries, while magnesium and phosphorus work to enhance the bone matrix's structural integrity.

The quest for these vital nutrients leads to diverse dietary sources, painting a picture of meals rich in color and texture. Leafy greens such as kale and spinach emerge as verdant treasures, offering calcium and vitamin K in generous portions. Fatty fish, basking in the glow of their vitamin D content, provide skeletal support and a heart-healthy dose of omega-3 fatty acids. Dairy products, fortified cereals, and plant-based milks are calcium bastions. At the same time, nuts, seeds, and whole grains bring magnesium into the fold. When strategically placed within the eating windows of intermittent fasting, this dietary diversification ensures a steady supply of bone-building nutrients, each meal a step toward sturdier, more resilient bones.

Yet, the narrative of bone health is not woven from diet alone but is influenced profoundly by the tapestry of lifestyle factors that paint the backdrop of daily life. Physical activity, particularly weight-bearing exercises, echoes the adage of "use it or lose it," stimulating bone formation and signaling the body to reinforce the skeletal framework. In measured doses, sun exposure acts as a catalyst for vitamin D synthesis; its rays coax the skin to produce this bone-protective nutrient. However, the modern lifestyle, marked by indoor living and sunscreen use, often casts a shadow on this natural process, necessitating a mindful approach to sun exposure and, in some cases, dietary supplementation to ensure adequate vitamin D levels.

Therefore, monitoring and managing bone health becomes an act of vigilance, a proactive stance against the encroaching threat of osteoporosis. Bone density scans, recommended at intervals by healthcare professionals, provide a glimpse into the skeletal depths, revealing the state of bone health and the effectiveness of dietary and lifestyle strategies. Adjustments to the diet, whether through the introduction of bone-building foods or the judicious use of supplements, become responsive maneuvers guided by the insights gleaned from these evaluations. This dynamic approach, attuned to the body's changing needs, ensures that the strategies employed are not static but evolve, mirroring the body's ongoing journey through the years.

In this intricate dance of nutrients, lifestyle choices, and proactive health management, the preservation of bone health emerges as a multifaceted endeavor. In this symphony, each element plays a critical role in the harmonious functioning of the whole. It is a narrative that unfolds daily, with each meal, each burst of sunlight, and each step taken a testament to the body's remarkable capacity for renewal and resilience. In this story, the choices made at the dining table, the dedication to physical activity, and the attentiveness to the body's signals converge, crafting a path toward enduring strength and vitality, ensuring that the bones that support us stand firm, not just in the face of advancing age but in the embrace of life itself.

PROTEIN INTAKE AND MUSCLE PRESERVATION

In the intricate dance of aging, where the body's once robust rhythms begin to slow, the role of protein ascends, assuming a pivotal position in maintaining muscle mass and overall vitality. This period, often marked by the hormonal shifts of menopause, witnesses a subtle yet significant erosion of muscle strength. This phenomenon not only impacts physical capability but also metabolic health. In this context, protein, in its myriad forms, emerges as a beacon of preservation, a nutrient capable of counteracting the relentless tide of muscle degradation that accompanies the advancing years.

Protein, the architect of the body's structural integrity, is the foundation upon which muscle fibers are built and repaired. Its importance burgeons during and after menopause, when the body's natural muscle preservation mechanisms wane under hormonal changes. The synthesis of new muscle protein, a process once brisk and efficient, becomes a labor of more deliberate pacing, necessitating an increased dietary protein intake to maintain muscle mass and strength. This heightened need underscores the necessity of identifying high-quality protein sources that can seamlessly integrate into women's nutritional patterns while navigating this transformative phase.

High-quality protein sources span a vast and varied landscape, from the verdant fields of plant-based options to the azure depths of the sea. For those whose dietary preferences lean toward the vegetarian or vegan, legumes, tofu, tempeh, and a diverse array of nuts and seeds stand as stalwarts of protein, each offering not just the building blocks of muscle but a constellation of other nutrients beneficial for health. When creatively incorporated into meals, these plant-based proteins ensure that the diet remains rich in essential amino acids and aligned with ethical and ecological values. For those who derive their sustenance from the sea and land, fish, poultry, and lean cuts of meat provide protein in its most bioavailable form, ensuring that the body's needs for muscle repair and growth are met with precision and ease.

Integrating protein into the eating windows defined by intermittent fasting necessitates intention and strategy. The goal is to distribute protein intake evenly across meals, a practice that optimizes muscle protein synthesis, ensuring that the body remains in a state of constant repair and renewal. Far from a mere logistical challenge, this distribution invites creativity in meal planning, where protein becomes the centerpiece around which other macronutrients and micronutrients gather. For breakfast, you might see a fusion of eggs and spinach; for lunch, a symphony of quinoa and black beans; and for dinner, a medley of salmon and asparagus. Snacks, too, become opportunities for protein enrichment, with Greek yogurt, cottage cheese, and a handful of almonds serving as both nourishment and pleasure.

Yet, the narrative of muscle preservation extends beyond the realm of nutrition into physical activity, where resistance training emerges as a powerful ally. This form of exercise, characterized by the lifting, pushing, or pulling of weight, acts as a catalyst for muscle growth, sending a clear signal to the body that strength is not just desired but demanded. The synergy between adequate protein intake and resistance training is profound, each reinforcing the other in a continuous improvement cycle. Protein provides the raw materials for muscle repair and growth. At the same time, resistance training ensures that these materials are utilized to their fullest potential, enhancing the body's functional ability and metabolic health.

This partnership, forged in the pursuit of muscle preservation, is not static but dynamic, evolving in response to the body's changing needs and capacities. It recognizes that resistance training, like protein intake, must be tailored to the individual, considering physical capabilities, preferences, and goals. It might manifest as bodyweight exercises performed in the living room, weights lifted in the peaceful ambiance of a gym, or resistance bands stretched in the privacy of a home office. The form matters less than the function, engaging the muscles in a deliberate and sustained effort to counteract the natural decline accompanying aging.

In this multifaceted approach to protein intake and muscle preservation, women over fifty find a strategy for maintaining physical strength and a blueprint for sustaining vitality. It is an approach that marries the nutritional with the physical, the dietary with the active, ensuring that the body remains a vessel for life and a vibrant and capable participant in it. Through the strategic consumption of high-quality protein and the deliberate practice of resistance training, the challenge of muscle preservation is met with determination and grace, ensuring that the advancing years are marked not by decline but by a deepened capacity for strength, resilience, and health.

MANAGING CRAVINGS AND MAKING HEALTHY SWAPS

Cravings, those insistent calls from our bodies that push us toward specific tastes, textures, or foods, hold a complex place within the tapestry of our dietary habits, especially during the transformative phase of menopause. These urges, often painted as mere whims of the appetite, in reality, stem from a confluence of physiological shifts and psychological states. The ebb and flow of hormones like estrogen, which dips during menopause, can significantly impact our sense of hunger and fullness, tilting the scales toward an increased propensity for cravings. This hormonal fluctuation, coupled with the body's natural inclination to seek comfort during periods of stress or emotional upheaval, positions cravings at the intersection of physical need and emotional longing.

In navigating these cravings, the concept of healthy swaps emerges as a strategy not of denial but of substitution, where the focus is on fulfilling these urges without diverging from the path of nutritional integrity. This approach requires a keen understanding of the craving—whether for something sweet, salty, or savory—and the underlying need it signifies. For the sweet tooth urged on by a drop in serotonin levels, a piece of dark chocolate, rich in flavor and antioxidants, can satisfy the craving while offering a mood lift. For the crunch and salt sought in moments of stress, air-popped popcorn seasoned with a dash of sea salt and nutritional yeast provides a satisfying alternative to the traditional, more indulgent options like potato chips.

The art of managing cravings extends into the realm of proactive meal and snack planning, a strategy that anticipates rather than reacts to the onset of cravings. This foresight involves assembling meals that balance macronutrients—proteins for satiety, carbohydrates for energy, and fats for flavor—thereby stabilizing blood sugar levels and warding off the sharp spikes and drops that can trigger cravings. Snack preparation plays a crucial role here, where having readily available, nutrient-dense options prevents the easy fallback to less healthful choices when hunger or cravings strike unexpectedly. This preparation, while practical, also serves as a ritual of self-care, a reminder of the importance of nourishing the body with intention and mindfulness.

Yet, beyond the physiological lies the realm of emotional eating, a landscape where cravings are not just signals of nutritional need but expressions of emotional states—boredom, loneliness, stress, or joy. Menopause, with its tapestry of physical and emotional changes, can amplify these states, making the draw of emotional eating more potent. In this context, managing cravings becomes an exercise in emotional awareness and regulation, where the first step is recognizing the emotional cue behind the craving. This recognition opens the door to alternative self-soothing forms, such as engaging in a hobby, taking a walk, practicing deep breathing, or connecting with a friend, each offering a way to fulfill the emotional need without turning to food.

Integrating these strategies—healthy swaps, proactive planning, and emotional awareness—into the fabric of daily life requires knowledge, resilience, patience, and a dose of creativity. It's a continuous learning and adapting process that acknowledges the dynamic nature of our bodies and needs. In this light, cravings are not adversaries to be defeated but signals to be understood, a dialogue between body and mind that enriches our relationship with food and ourselves when approached with curiosity and compassion.

THE TRUTH ABOUT CARBS: FRIEND OR FOE?

In the vast landscape of nutritional discourse, carbohydrates stand at a crossroads, heralded by some as the cornerstone of a balanced diet and maligned by others as the root of all dietary evil. For women navigating the intricate shifts of their fifties, understanding the true nature of carbohydrates is akin to deciphering a complex code, one that, when cracked, illuminates the path to sustained energy and health. The vilification of carbohydrates has woven a narrative fraught with oversimplifications. However, beneath the surface lies a nuanced story of diversity, where the distinction between complex and simple forms of carbohydrates holds the key to unlocking their true potential.

Carbohydrates, in their essence, are the body's primary source of fuel, a collection of sugars, starches, and fibers that furnish the energy required for everything from cerebral functions to muscular contractions. Yet, not all carbohydrates are created equal, which becomes pivotal in distinguishing those that nourish from those that merely satiate. Complex carbohydrates, characterized by their long chains of sugar molecules, offer a sustained release of energy. Their gradual digestion ensures a steady fuel supply that mitigates the sharp spikes and troughs in blood sugar levels synonymous with their simpler counterparts. These complex forms, found abundantly in whole grains, legumes, and a wealth of vegetables, also come replete with fibers, vitamins, and minerals, enhancing their stature as nutritional powerhouses.

The narrative takes a divergent path when the spotlight shifts to simple carbohydrates with shorter sugar chains that offer a rapid but fleeting burst of energy. Often hidden within processed foods and sugary confections, these carbohydrates flirt with the body's metabolic balance, eliciting swift rises in blood sugar levels followed by equally rapid declines. This cycle can fray the body's energetic equilibrium and, over time, wear down its insulin responsiveness. This dichotomy between complex and simple carbohydrates forms the crux of understanding how to harness their potential without succumbing to their pitfalls.

Enter the glycemic index (GI) and glycemic load (GL), tools designed to measure the impact of carbohydrates on blood sugar levels. The GI ranks carbohydrates on a scale from 0 to 100 based on how quickly they raise blood sugar levels after eating. At the same time, the GL refines this measure by accounting for the amount of carbohydrates in a portion of food. Foods with a low GI and GL are slow to impact blood sugar levels, offering a moderated energy release that aligns with the body's natural rhythms. Incorporating these low GI and GL foods into the eating windows of intermittent fasting becomes a strategic move, ensuring that the body is fueled by a steady energy source that complements the fasting-induced metabolic adjustments.

The dance between carbohydrates and intermittent fasting is delicate, a ballet where timing, quantity, and quality converge. Within the confines of eating windows, prioritizing complex carbohydrates becomes a strategic endeavor, ensuring that every meal is not just a moment of nourishment but a building block in health architecture. These meals, rich in fibers and nutrients, do more than satiate; they sustain, offering the body a reservoir of energy that endures through the fasting periods, ensuring that hunger pangs are kept at bay and energy levels remain buoyant.

Yet, the tale of carbohydrates is not confined to the realm of nutrition science but extends into the domain of culinary arts, where the simple act of choosing whole-grain bread over its white counterpart or opting for a serving of quinoa instead of white rice transforms the mundane into the extraordinary. It's in the vibrancy of a meal adorned with legumes, the satisfaction derived from a bowl brimming with leafy greens, and the comfort found in a serving of oatmeal that the true essence of carbohydrates is revealed. This essence lies not in the quantity but in the quality, not in the avoidance but in the intelligent selection and integration of carbohydrates into the diet.

In closing, the journey through carbohydrates, particularly for women over fifty, is not a path of avoidance but an enlightened choice. It's a journey where complex carbohydrates become trusted allies, their incorporation into the eating windows of intermittent fasting a testament to the power of informed dietary decisions. As this chapter draws closer, we are reminded of the broader nutrition narrative. In this narrative, balance, variety, and moderation are pillars of health and vitality. With this understanding, we turn our gaze forward, ready to explore the next chapter in our quest for well-being, armed with the knowledge that in the world of nutrition, as in life, the truth often lies in the balance.

HELP OTHERS MAKE ONE VITAL DECISION THAT COULD REVOLUTIONIZE THEIR HEALTH

If you do not change direction, you may end up where you are heading.

— LAO TZU

At the very start of this book, I mentioned the positive effects of intermittent fasting on autophagy, insulin sensitivity improvement, and the rise in growth hormone levels. It is truly amazing to think that a lifestyle that is so easy to adopt can have such a profound impact on your body and mind.

You may have developed an interest in intermittent fasting as a means to curb hot flashes or battle weight gain, but the benefits it brings not only improve menopausal symptoms, but also have the ability to lengthen your lifespan. Indeed, anyone who wishes to transform their body into a well-oiled, energetic, balanced machine can benefit from the practice of fasting.

Thus far, you have seen the cascade of advantages that intermittent fasting brings, including stabilizing estrogen and progesterone levels. You have also discovered that it is a powerful tool in the battle against stress. If what you've read has helped you change your outlook on life for the better, then I hope you can spread the word to those who are ready to embrace holistic change… the kind that will stand them in good stead as they move through menopause and beyond.

By leaving a short review on Amazon, you'll let other readers know that intermittent fasting isn't a fad or a mere weight loss

regimen. It is a lifestyle choice that works on multiple levels to enhance your physical and mental health.

By letting others know how the strategies in this book worked for you, you may inspire them to make lasting changes. There are so many misconceptions about intermittent fasting, including the idea that you need to go hungry or suffer to see results. You can debunk those myths simply by sharing a little bit about yourself and your experiences with IF.

Thanks for your support. Together, we can end the reign of insulin resistance in one fell swoop.

Scan the QR code below:

MEAL MASTERY DURING YOUR FASTING WINDOW

Navigating the waters of intermittent fasting reveals a landscape rich with the potential for transformation, where the rhythm of fasting and feeding frames our days, and the choices made within these sacred intervals dictate the trajectory of our health. The alchemy of nutrition unfolds within the confines of these feeding windows, an ancient and profoundly personal process where the foods we select become the materials from which our bodies are continually reborn. Here, amid the ebb and flow of fasting, lies an opportunity for restraint and abundance, a time to nourish, replenish, and delight in the bounty that food offers.

CREATING A 28-DAY INTERMITTENT FASTING MEAL PLAN

Structured Flexibility

A 28-day meal plan serves as a compass, guiding through the terrain of intermittent fasting with precision yet allowing for detours that accommodate the unpredictability of life. Imagine planning a garden; some seeds need planting at specific times, yet weather and wildlife will influence the garden's yield. Similarly, this meal plan combines structured eating times with the flexibility to adjust to late meetings, family gatherings, or the simple desire for variety. The plan, laid out weekly, allocates specific windows for eating, interspersed with recipes that cater to diverse palates and nutritional needs, ensuring that every plate is a mosaic of color, texture, and taste.

Nutritional Balance

Each meal within this plan is a testament to balance, designed to meet the nutritional demands peculiar to women over fifty. Calcium for bone density, iron to fend off anemia, and omega-3 fatty acids for brain health form the cornerstone of this nutritional edifice. Visualize a plate divided into quarters: one half filled with vibrant greens and colorful vegetables, a quarter with lean protein, and the remaining quarter with whole grains or starchy vegetables, a visual guide ensuring that each meal is a holistic representation of the needed macronutrients and micronutrients.

Prep and Planning Tips

The art of meal prep is akin to setting the stage for a performance, where each ingredient plays its part to perfection. On a Sunday afternoon, consider dedicating a couple of hours to prepare the staples: grains cooked and stored, proteins marinated and perhaps partially cooked, and vegetables washed and chopped. Much like rehearsing a play, this preparation ensures that the scene unfolds quickly when the curtain rises at mealtime, reducing the temptation to deviate toward less nourishing choices.

Adaptability

No matter how meticulously crafted, a meal plan must possess the quality of water, be able to flow around obstacles and adapt to the container of our daily lives. This plan offers alternatives for those navigating dietary restrictions, whether by choice or necessity: plant-based proteins stand in for animal products, gluten-free grains replace their wheat-based counterparts, and dairy alternatives offer richness without lactose. Therefore, each recipe within the plan comes with a sidebar of swaps, ensuring that the meal plan is not a rigid framework but a fluid guide that respects and accommodates individual dietary landscapes.

Textual Element: Your 28-Day Intermittent Fasting Blueprint

A checklist emerges as a tangible tool, a blueprint laying the foundation for four weeks of nourished fasting:

- Week 1 Focus: Ease into fasting with simple, nutrient-dense meals. Start with familiar favorites, gradually introducing new ingredients.

- Week 2 Exploration: Experiment with one new recipe or ingredient each day. Note reactions, preferences, and any energy changes.
- Week 3 Consolidation: Identify and replicate the most satisfying meals, adjusting portions and ingredients as needed.
- Week 4 Reflection: Review the past weeks. Which meals provided the most energy? Which felt lacking? Adjust the plan based on these insights.

The goal in crafting this 28-day meal plan transcends mere sustenance; it is about creating a tapestry of meals that nourish, satisfy, and inspire. It is a journey through the world of flavors and nutrients, a deliberate practice that marries the science of nutrition with the art of cooking, ensuring that each meal within the fasting window becomes a stepping stone toward health, vitality, and joy.

Your 28-Day Intermittent Fasting Meal Plan

General Daily Eating Pattern

- Breakfast (Start of 8-hour eating window): Aim for a balance of protein, healthy fats, and fiber to keep you feeling satisfied.
- Lunch: Include a variety of vegetables, lean protein, and whole grains for energy and nutrients.
- Snack (Optional): Choose nutrient-dense options like nuts, seeds, yogurt, or fruit.
- Dinner (End of 8-hour eating window): Focus on lean protein and vegetables, with moderate healthy fats to promote satiety throughout the fasting period.

Week 1: Introduction

Day 1:

- Breakfast: Greek yogurt with mixed berries and a handful of walnuts.
- Lunch: Quinoa salad with grilled chicken, mixed greens, cucumbers, tomatoes, and avocado, dressed with olive oil and lemon juice.
- Snack: A small apple with almond butter.
- Dinner: Baked salmon with asparagus and a side of wild rice.

Repeat variations of Day 1 for Days 2–7, adjusting protein sources (e.g., tofu, lentils, fish, chicken), types of berries and nuts, and swapping different vegetables and whole grains in meals to ensure variety and nutrient coverage.

Week 2: Establishing Routine

Day 8:

- Breakfast: Scrambled eggs with spinach, mushrooms, and feta cheese.
- Lunch: Turkey and hummus wrap with whole grain tortilla, mixed greens, shredded carrots, and bell peppers.
- Snack: Greek yogurt with a sprinkle of chia seeds.
- Dinner: Grilled shrimp over mixed leafy greens with quinoa, avocado, and cherry tomatoes, dressed with a vinaigrette.

Continue with similar variations for Days 9–14, focusing on mixing up the types of lean proteins, vegetables, and grains.

Week 3: Nutritional Focus

Day 15:

- Breakfast: Overnight oats with almond milk, chia seeds, mixed berries, and a dash of honey.
- Lunch: Lentil soup with a side salad of mixed greens, cucumber, and a few slices of avocado.
- Snack: Carrot sticks with hummus.
- Dinner: Stir-fried tofu with broccoli, bell peppers, and snap peas over brown rice.

Days 16–21 should continue to focus on plant-based proteins, whole grains, and a colorful array of vegetables, adjusting recipes to include a variety of nutrients.

Week 4: Diverse and Mindful Eating

Day 22:

- Breakfast: Smoothie with spinach, banana, protein powder, almond milk, and a tablespoon of flaxseed.
- Lunch: Chickpea salad with cherry tomatoes, cucumber, olives, feta, and quinoa.
- Snack: A peach and a handful of almonds.
- Dinner: Grilled chicken with a mixed vegetable medley (zucchini, eggplant, bell pepper) and a side of farro.

For Days 23–28, encourage experimentation with different fruits, vegetables, whole grains, and protein sources to keep meals interesting and nutritionally balanced.

Notes

- Hydration is crucial; drink water throughout the day, especially during fasting periods.
- Adjust portion sizes according to individual needs and satiety cues.
- Before starting any new diet, especially for women over fifty with unique nutritional needs, consulting with a healthcare provider or a dietitian is recommended.

This plan is a starting point meant to inspire a balanced and varied diet that complements an intermittent fasting lifestyle. Adjust as necessary to fit personal health needs, preferences, and goals.

QUICK AND NUTRITIOUS RECIPES FOR BUSY WOMEN

In the whirl of day-to-day responsibilities, where hours compress and expand in unexpected rhythms, finding solace in the kitchen becomes both a challenge and a necessity. For the woman who strides with purpose through the corridors of her career, tends to the family's needs, and still seeks moments of personal enrichment, preparing a meal transcends the mundane; it becomes a quiet assertion of self-care amid the din of daily obligations. Thus, the need for recipes that marry nutrition with convenience arises —not as a compromise but as a celebration of efficiency and health.

Time-Saving Recipes

Imagine dishes that come together with the grace of a well-rehearsed dance, where each step and ingredient seamlessly blends into the next, culminating in meals that nourish as much as they delight. A smoothie, vibrant with the hues of spinach, berries, and a dash of protein powder, offers a morning ritual that awakens the senses and the mind. Soups, rich with legumes, lean meats, and an abundance of vegetables, simmer to perfection with minimal attendance, their flavors deepening as they await the dinner hour. Sheet pan dinners, where proteins and vegetables roast in unison, create symphonies of flavor with the simplicity of a single pan. These recipes, curated with the precision of a timekeeper, ensure that nourishment is never sacrificed at the altar of haste.

Batch Cooking

The strategy of batch cooking emerges as a beacon for those navigating the tight shoals of time. By dedicating a few hours on a weekend to preparing meals for the week, one transforms time from foe to ally. This practice, akin to laying in provisions before a voyage, ensures that the week ahead is navigated with the assurance of wholesome meals ready. Imagine a cauldron of chili, its spices melding over the slow passage of hours, or trays of roasted vegetables, their edges caramelizing to a sweet complexity. Once portioned and stored, these provisions become the keystones of meals that assemble with the ease of a sigh, turning the potential stress of mealtime into an oasis of calm.

Ingredient Swaps

In the alchemy of cooking, the substitution of ingredients serves not merely as a tactic for addressing absent pantry items but as a strategy for enhancing nutritional content without diluting flavor or intention. A purée of white beans stands in for cream, lending silkiness to soups and sauces while boosting protein and fiber. Cauliflower, when riced, becomes a chameleon, adept at replacing grains for those navigating the complexities of carbohydrate management. Zucchini ribbons twirl with the promise of pasta, yet they carry a lighter burden of calories and a bounty of nutrients. Through these swaps, meals retain their allure and satisfaction, even as their compositions shift to align with health goals and dietary preferences.

Kitchen Staples

The foundation of quick, nutritious cooking lies in the arsenal of ingredients at one's disposal. Stocking the pantry and fridge with staples ensures that meal preparation is not a constant negotiation with time and availability but a fluid extension of daily routine. Quinoa and brown rice, with their generous profiles of protein and fiber, offer a ready base for an array of dishes, from salads to stir-fries. Cans of rinsed and drained legumes stand ready to bolster soups, salads, and even desserts with their hearty substance. A rainbow of spices, from the smoky depth of paprika to the bright zing of lemon pepper, promises to elevate the simplest ingredients into culinary delights. In the cool recesses of the fridge, a collection of Greek yogurts, mixed greens, and an assortment of fresh vegetables await their turn to grace the plate, each bringing its own spectrum of flavors and nutrients.

Proper storage extends the freshness and utility of these staples. Grains, when stored in airtight containers, shrug off the threat of moisture and pests. Vegetables, nestled in the crisper with an understanding of their unique humidity needs, retain their crispness and vitality. Herbs, washed and stored carefully, lend their aromatic notes to dishes long after purchase.

In this landscape of quick, nutritious recipes, batch cooking, savvy ingredient swaps, and well-stocked pantries, the preparation of meals transforms from a task to be managed into an act of grace and creativity. It becomes a space where health and flavor fuse, where time constraints are met with ingenuity and foresight, ensuring that even on the busiest days, nourishment remains a constant, unwavering companion on the journey of wellness and vitality.

PREPPING MEALS FOR SUCCESS

A well-thought-out strategy becomes indispensable in the meticulous choreography of meal preparation that aligns with intermittent fasting schedules. Here, the objective is not merely to fill the pantry with wholesome ingredients but to ensure that every dish crafted not only satiates but also enriches, transforming eating into a nourishing ritual. This process, while intricate, offers a canvas on which patterns of healthy eating are painted, each stroke deliberate, each hue vibrant with nutrients, ensuring that the body's needs are met with precision during those critical eating windows.

Meal Prep Strategies

Embarking on this path requires a map—a detailed plan that anticipates needs, preferences, and the unpredictable currents of daily life. It begins with a survey of the week ahead, noting the rhythm of work commitments, social engagements, and moments of solitude. Against this backdrop, meals are plotted, each chosen for its ability to offer sustenance and pleasure without demanding undue time or effort in the kitchen. The strategy embraces the grandeur of diversity and the comfort of routine, alternating between tried-and-true favorites and new culinary explorations, ensuring that the palate remains engaged and the body well-nourished. Once in place, this plan serves as a guide, flexible enough to accommodate the ebb and flow of appetite and schedule yet structured sufficiently to prevent the drift into less healthful choices.

Tools and Equipment

The arsenal for this culinary endeavor is carefully selected, each utensil and appliance a chosen ally in the quest for efficiency and effectiveness. High-speed blenders stand ready to transform fruits and greens into smoothies, imbuing the morning with vibrancy. Slow cookers simmer ingredients to perfection, their contents a promise of hearty meals awaiting at the day's end. Quality knives glide through vegetables and meats, their sharpness preserving the integrity of each slice. At the same time, a set of durable, nonstick pans ensures that cooking surfaces require minimal oil, allowing the natural flavors of food to take center stage. While varied, this selection of tools and equipment shares a common purpose: to simplify the meal preparation process, making it manageable and enjoyable.

Mindful Portioning

Within meal prep, portioning emerges as a critical skill, a means to calibrate intake with need, ensuring that each meal fits within the parameters of dietary goals without tipping into excess. This skill requires understanding nutritional requirements, sensitivity to the body's cues, and the ability to gauge satiety and satisfaction. Containers of various sizes become the vessels through which portions are measured, each filled with a balance of macronutrients—proteins for muscle repair, carbohydrates for energy, and fats for satiety and flavor. This process, though methodical, is imbued with a sense of care, a recognition that each container holds not just food but fuel for life's endeavors.

Storing and Reheating

The final act in this prelude to nourishment is the preservation of meals, ensuring freshness and flavor are locked in, ready to be released upon reheating. The science of storage is precise, requiring an understanding of temperature, air exposure, and the delicate balance of moisture that can either preserve or spoil. Glass containers, with their inert surfaces, offer a sanctuary for prepped meals, their transparency a window into the colors and textures of stored dishes. Refrigeration is calibrated, with settings adjusted to maintain an optimal environment for preservation. The reheating process, too, is approached with care, with methods chosen to restore warmth and texture without compromising nutritional integrity. Microwaves, when used, are set to medium power to avoid overheating. At the same time, stovetop and oven reheating are preferred for dishes where crispness and texture are paramount.

In this meticulous orchestration of meal prep, the goal transcends mere sustenance; it is an endeavor that seeks to infuse each eating window with intention and care, ensuring that the body is not only fed but truly nourished. Through strategic planning, carefully selecting tools and equipment, mindful portioning, and attentive storage and reheating, meal preparation becomes an integral part of the fasting journey, a testament to the commitment to health and well-being that guides each choice, each dish, and each bite.

EATING OUT AND SOCIAL EVENTS: STAYING ON TRACK

The terrain shifts in the intricate dance of social engagements and the ritual of dining beyond the confines of one's kitchen. Here, amid the conviviality of shared meals and celebrating milestones, the principles guiding intermittent fasting and nutritional choices face their sternest test. This test, however, is not a skirmish to be won or lost in a single evening but a series of choices that reflect a more profound commitment to well-being, balanced against the joy and spontaneity that social connections bring.

Navigating Menus

Perusing a menu, whether scrolled on a chalkboard or elegantly printed, becomes an exercise in discernment. It's a moment to pause, to scan not just for what tantalizes the palate but for options that align with the nourishment one seeks within one's eating window. Opting for dishes that spotlight lean proteins and an abundance of vegetables, seasoned with herbs and spices over heavy sauces, can transform a meal into an extension of one's nutritional regimen without veering into asceticism. In this, the dialogue with servers becomes pivotal, and their insights into the menu's offerings are a resource to be leveraged for making choices that satisfy both the senses and the dietary ethos one follows.

Communicating Dietary Preferences

In the warmth of a friend's dining room or the laughter-filled ambiance of a social gathering, the challenge often lies not in the availability of fasting-friendly options but in articulating one's dietary preferences. This articulation, far from a demand placed upon hosts, is a gentle negotiation, a sharing of one's commitment to health that invites accommodation rather than imposes constraints. Offering to bring a dish that complements the meal yet stays true to one's dietary principles serves a dual purpose: it eases the burden on the host while ensuring that the meal aligns with one's nutritional path. This approach fosters an atmosphere of inclusivity and respect, where dietary choices are shared and celebrated rather than hidden or apologized for.

Mindful Indulgence

Amid the clinking of glasses and the shared laughter over a sumptuous spread, indulgence beckons; it whispers of the richness of life, of the pleasure found in a bite of a decadent dessert or the sip of a fine wine. To indulge mindfully is to walk the tightrope between deprivation and excess, finding a middle ground where the moment's joy is savored without the shadow of regret. It's choosing the slice of cake but forgoing the second, allowing the sweetness to linger on the tongue, and, in the memory, a momentary departure from the norm rather than a derailing of one's dietary journey. This delicate and personal balance underscores the importance of presence, of fully inhabiting the moment and the choice, making indulgence a part of the journey rather than an escape.

Strategies for Success

As the calendar fills with invitations, navigating these social waters demands foresight. Pre-event, a smaller meal that balances proteins and fibers can mitigate the edge of hunger, reducing the temptation to overindulge upon arrival. Hydration, too, becomes a shield, warding off the false hunger that thirst often masquerades as. At the heart of the event, plate selection offers a canvas on which to paint one's meal with intention. Starting with vegetables, adding proteins, and then considering grains or more indulgent options creates a visual and nutritional balance that satisfies without overtaxing the digestive system. Above all, the focus remains on the people, the conversation, and the shared experiences that are the proper nourishment these gatherings offer. In this, the act of eating becomes a part of the social fabric, woven into the evening's tapestry rather than standing apart as a challenge to be navigated.

In these moments, the journey of intermittent fasting and nutritional mindfulness reveals its true nature: not as a path of restriction but as a framework within which the fullness of life can be embraced. It underscores the possibility of balance, of finding a way to celebrate, to connect, and to indulge without losing sight of the commitment to one's health and well-being. This balance achieved not through rigidity but through the fluidity of choice and the clarity of intention, becomes a testament to the possibility of living entirely within the structures we set for ourselves, a dance of discipline and delight that enriches both the body and the spirit.

THE ROLE OF MINDFUL EATING IN INTERMITTENT FASTING

Within the framework of intermittent fasting, where the temporal boundaries of consumption are defined, mindful eating emerges as a beacon, illuminating the path to a deeper understanding of the body's signals and fostering a relationship with food that transcends mere sustenance. This approach, rooted in presence and awareness, encourages communion with each bite, reverence for the nourishment provided, and attunement to the body's innate wisdom.

Enhancing Awareness

In the quiet spaces between fasting and feeding, mindful eating cultivates an acute sensitivity to the body's hunger cues and fullness. This heightened awareness guides the eater toward choices that resonate with the body's genuine needs rather than the whims of transient cravings or the allure of emotional eating. It is an invitation to listen, truly listen, to the whispers and roars of the body, discerning the difference between the need for nourishment and the desire for comfort or distraction. While simple in concept, this practice requires shedding preconceived notions and judgments about food and eating, allowing for an enriching and enlightening experience.

Eating without Distraction

In a world awash with stimuli, where meals are often consumed in tandem with screen time or amid the din of daily life, mindful eating advocates for a return to simplicity. It posits that meals should be unencumbered by distraction, allowing for a complete immersion in the experience of eating. This solitude is not born of isolation but of a desire to fully engage with nourishment, where food's textures, flavors, and aromas can be appreciated without the veil of external interference. In this undistracted state, eating slowly becomes not a chore but a natural rhythm, where satiety is reached with a satisfaction that transcends the physical and touches on the spiritual.

Savoring Flavors

The act of savoring, allowing each flavor and texture to unfold and reveal itself, is an art honed through mindful eating. It is a slow dance, a deliberate exploration of the nuances that each ingredient brings to the palate. This savoring does more than enhance the pleasure of eating; it serves as a counterbalance to the impulse to overeat, providing fulfillment that is not solely dependent on volume. Techniques such as chewing thoroughly, placing utensils down between bites, and pausing to reflect on the flavors transform eating from a mundane task into a rich sensory experience. Through this practice, meals become a tapestry of tastes and textures, each bite a thread, contributing to the overall masterpiece of the dining experience.

Emotional Connection

At the heart of mindful eating lies the unraveling of the emotional entanglements that often bind individuals to their eating patterns. Food is a source of energy and life in its most primal form. Yet, its role extends into comfort, celebration, and, sometimes, solace. Mindful eating invites an introspection into these emotional connections, offering a space to acknowledge and address the feelings that prompt eating outside the boundaries of hunger. It encourages the exploration of alternative avenues for emotional fulfillment, suggesting that while food can be a source of joy, it need not be the sole comforter. In recognizing these patterns, individuals forge a new relationship with food that respects its role as a nourisher while acknowledging the wealth of emotional experiences that life offers beyond the plate.

In integrating mindful eating into intermittent fasting, nourishment becomes a ritual, a sacred space carved out within the day where the focus is on the quality of the eating experience rather than the quantity of consumption. This approach fosters a harmony between body and mind, where food is both a pleasure and a source of sustenance, and eating is an act of self-respect and care. Through this lens, intermittent fasting transcends its boundaries as a dietary framework. It becomes a pathway to a more attuned, aware, and fulfilling way of eating and living.

SUCCESS STORIES: REAL WOMEN, REAL RESULTS

Within the tapestries of lives metamorphosed by the gentle yet persistent embrace of intermittent fasting and mindful nutrition, stories of women over fifty blossoms are a testament to the transformative power of dedication and insight. These narratives, rich in diversity and depth, weave a collective wisdom, a beacon for those navigating the nuanced path to wellness in the latter chapters of their lives.

Martha, a librarian from the coastal town of Maine, discovered intermittent fasting in the aftermath of a health scare that left her contemplating her mortality. Her journey began not with grand ambitions but with the modest hope of reclaiming her health, one meal at a time. Through the 16/8 method, Martha found not just a structure for eating but a new rhythm for living that harmonized her body's needs with the demands of her spirit. Her transformation, marked by a loss of twenty pounds and a newfound vibrancy, is a testament to persistence's power. Martha's lesson is simple yet profound: start small, stay consistent, and the body will return to health.

In contrast, Rachel's foray into intermittent fasting was driven by curiosity, a desire to explore the boundaries of her body's capabilities. A retired professional athlete, Rachel's transition from the rigor of training to the quieter pace of retirement left her searching for a method to maintain her fitness without the extremes of her past. Intermittent fasting, coupled with mindful nutrition, became her arena. In this space, she experimented with eating windows and nutrient-dense foods to find the balance that fit her new lifestyle. Her success, a blend of maintained muscle mass and enhanced energy levels, underscores the adaptability of intermittent fasting to cater to varied lifestyles and goals. From

Rachel, the insight gleaned is flexibility; the most effective fasting plan evolves with changing tides.

Then there's Anita, whose introduction to intermittent fasting came through the pages of a magazine. This lucky find piqued her interest during a time of personal upheaval. For Anita, fasting became a cornerstone of a broader endeavor to overhaul her life, from her nutrition to her physical activity and mental health. The community she found, both online and in her local yoga class, provided guidance and a sense of belonging—a reminder that the journey to wellness is best traveled with allies. Anita's story illuminates the role of community support in sustaining motivation, highlighting the strength of shared experiences and collective wisdom.

Each narrative, distinct in its contours, converges on a singular truth: that the journey to health, especially for women over fifty, is as much about nourishing the soul as it is about the body. The lessons these stories impart—of starting slightly, embracing flexibility, and leaning on community—form a triad of principles guiding wellness. They remind us that intermittent fasting and mindful nutrition are not just strategies for weight management or metabolic health but pathways to a fuller, more vibrant life.

In weaving these stories into the fabric of our understanding, we find not just inspiration but actionable wisdom—a compass to navigate our health journeys. It's in the sharing of these experiences that we find strength. This collective resilience encourages us to pursue our wellness goals with confidence and purpose. The tapestry of success stories, rich with the threads of real women achieving actual results, is a testament to the transformative power of intermittent fasting and mindful nutrition, offering a roadmap for those ready to embark on their journey to health and vitality.

As this chapter concludes, we are reminded of the intricate dance between body and spirit, a harmony achieved through the thoughtful embrace of intermittent fasting and mindful nutrition. These practices, grounded in the wisdom of real women's experiences, guide navigating the later years with grace and vigor. The stories shared here, each a beacon of possibility, illuminate the path forward, inviting us to explore the next chapter in our journey to wellness with open hearts and minds, ready to embrace the lessons and joys.

Amid the rhythm of daily life, where the ticking clock dictates the cadence of our actions, there exists a silent undercurrent, a force that propels us toward vitality and wellness. This force, often overlooked in the pursuit of dietary perfection, is exercise—a cornerstone of health that, when aligned with the body's needs and lifestyle, unfolds myriad benefits, extending far beyond the confines of physical well-being. In this nuanced exploration of movement, we delve into the symbiosis between exercise and intermittent fasting, unraveling the threads that weave together to form a tapestry of enduring vitality.

FINDING THE RIGHT EXERCISE FOR YOUR BODY AND LIFESTYLE

Personalization Is Key

Identifying exercises that resonate with one's interests and physical condition is akin to selecting the perfect pair of shoes; comfort, fit, and style are paramount, ensuring a willingness to wear them and enjoyment in their use. For exercise to become a woven part of one's daily fabric, it must echo personal preferences while accommodating physical limitations. This alignment fosters sustainability, transforming exercise from a task into a cherished part of one's routine. Imagine the difference between walking in a pair of well-fitted sneakers, feeling each step buoyed by comfort and support versus the discomfort of an ill-fitting pair; so, too, does the right exercise choice propel us forward with ease.

Low-Impact Options

For many, especially those navigating the physical considerations that often accompany life after fifty, low-impact exercises offer a sanctuary. These gentle yet effective activities promise the benefits of movement without the strain on joints and muscles that high-impact exercises might provoke. Walking, swimming, and cycling are beacons of low-impact exercise, each adaptable to varying fitness levels while offering the cardiovascular and muscular benefits essential for health. The accessibility of these exercises ensures that the door to physical activity remains open, inviting participation without fear of injury or undue stress.

Consistency over Intensity

In exercise, a whisper often carries more weight than a shout; so does the principle of consistency over intensity in crafting a routine that nurtures long-term health. While tempting, the allure of high-intensity sessions pales compared to the sustainable benefits of regular, moderate activity. This preference for steady, consistent effort over sporadic bursts of intensity underpins the development of a fitness routine that accommodates the realities of daily life and promotes enduring health benefits. It's the daily walks, the routine swims, and the regular cycles that compound over time, building a foundation of fitness that supports the body's evolving needs.

Incorporating Variety

Monotony is the nemesis of motivation, a truth that holds as much weight in exercise as it does in life. Infusing variety into one's exercise regimen is a balm for boredom, ensuring that interest remains piqued and engagement high. By rotating activities, from the meditative strokes of swimming to the rhythmic strides of walking, the body is challenged in new ways, preventing the plateau effect often seen with repetitive routines. This diversity caters to the body's comprehensive needs—addressing cardiovascular health, flexibility, and strength—and keeps the mind engaged, making exercise an anticipated part of the day rather than a mundane task.

Textual Element: Your Exercise Blueprint

A checklist emerges as a practical guide for integrating exercise into the fabric of life, ensuring that movement becomes a thread that strengthens the overall tapestry of wellness:

- Daily Movement Goals: Set achievable daily goals that encourage movement, whether a 30-minute walk or a 10-minute stretching session.
- Interest Inventory: List activities you enjoy alongside those you want to try. Use this as a roadmap for incorporating variety into your routine.
- Physical Assessment: Note any physical limitations or concerns, crafting your exercise plan to accommodate these considerations and ensure safety and comfort.
- Progress Journal: Keep a journal of your activities, reflecting on how each session felt, what you enjoyed, and how your body and mind responded.

In the gentle interplay between exercise and intermittent fasting, harmony is found—a balance that nurtures the body and the spirit. Through the thoughtful selection of activities that resonate with personal interests and physical capabilities, the embrace of low-impact options, a commitment to consistency, and the infusion of variety, exercise transcends its physical bounds, becoming a pillar of vitality and wellness. This movement journey, each step, stroke, and cycle, is a testament to the enduring power of exercise, a force that, when harnessed with intention and care, cultivates a life of vitality, strength, and joy.

STRENGTH TRAINING: THE KEY TO MUSCLE AND BONE HEALTH

In the intricate lattice that constitutes our bodily framework, muscle, and bone are the pillars upon which our physical prowess and metabolic vitality rest. Within this context, strength training emerges not merely as an activity relegated to those seeking aesthetic enhancement but as a fundamental practice for those intent on safeguarding their musculoskeletal integrity against the relentless tide of time. This section unfolds how resistance training acts as a bulwark, preserving muscle mass and bone density and equipping individuals with the strength and endurance necessary for life's demands.

Building Muscle Mass

The process of accruing muscle mass through strength training is not merely an endeavor of physical transformation but a critical measure for metabolic health maintenance. Each contraction, from lifting a dumbbell to resisting a band, signals the muscle fibers to fortify. This response transcends the visible hypertrophy to encompass enhancements in metabolic rate, insulin sensitivity, and even cognitive function. The cascade of benefits that emanates from this muscular engagement underscores the role of strength training as a catalyst, igniting a series of physiological adaptations that bolster the body against the insidious encroachments of age and sedentary living. Once dormant in their complacency, the fibers awaken, weaving a denser, more resilient fabric of musculature that burns calories with an efficiency that belies the simplicity of its activation.

Protecting Bone Density

Parallel to the fortification of muscle is the preservation of bone density, a critical concern as the calendar pages turn. Resistance exercises, in their myriad forms, from the press of a leg against the weight to the pull of a row, exert a stress upon the skeletal system that it cannot help but answer. This stress, far from detrimental, is a clarion call to the osteoblasts, urging them to lay down new bone and reinforce the architecture that underpins our ability to stand, move, and live. The dialogue between muscle and bone, mediated by resistance strain, becomes a fortress against osteoporosis. This shield guards our mobility and independence fiercely.

Equipment and Techniques

The armamentarium required for this endeavor can be simple and expansive; instead, the precision in selection and application dictates the efficacy of strength training. Dumbbells, kettlebells, resistance bands, and even one's body weight are sentinels, each offering a unique path to muscular engagement. With its versatility, the dumbbell invites a symphony of movements that challenge the muscles from every conceivable angle—kettlebells, with their off-center mass, demand stabilization, a co-conspirator in the quest for functional strength—resistance bands' tension variable and footprint minimal, offer a portability that belies their potency. And the body, an apparatus unto itself, when leveraged through push-ups, squats, and planks, becomes the medium through which strength is tested and gained. As critical as the tool, the technique hinges on the alignment of form with function, ensuring that each movement is executed with a mindfulness that maximizes benefit while minimizing risk.

Safety First

The initiation of a strength training regimen, especially for those at the juncture of midlife and beyond, is an exercise in prudence. The paramountcy of safety cannot be overstated; it is the lens through which all activity should be viewed and evaluated. Proper form, the cornerstone of safe practice, ensures that each exercise has an alignment that respects the body's natural mechanics, reducing the likelihood of strain or injury. Pacing is a critical consideration, a reminder that accumulating strength is a marathon, not a sprint. The incremental increase of weight or resistance, guided by the body's feedback, fosters a progression that is both sustainable and responsive to the individual's evolving capabilities. In this careful calibration of activity, the risk is mitigated, allowing the benefits of strength training to be reaped without the shadow of harm.

In physical well-being, where diet and exercise dance in a perpetual pas de deux, strength training stands as a pillar, supporting not just the body's form but its function. The dialogue between muscle and bone, facilitated by the deliberate application of stress and resistance, crafts a bastion against the decline, a testament to the body's remarkable capacity for renewal and resilience. Through the judicious selection and application of equipment and techniques, underscored by an unwavering commitment to safety, strength training transcends its physical bounds, becoming a conduit for a vitality that endures, a force that empowers individuals to navigate the complexities of life with strength, grace, and vigor.

GENTLE MOBILITY WORKOUTS AND THEIR BENEFITS

In the tapestry of physical wellness, where strength and endurance often capture the spotlight, gentle mobility workouts' subtle yet profound benefits weave their own intricate pattern. These practices, encompassing movements designed to cultivate flexibility, stand not as mere exercises in bending and stretching but as critical components in maintaining bodily harmony and preventing injury. The adoption of such routines into one's life serves not just to enhance physical capabilities but to foster a deeper connection between mind and body. In this symbiosis, movement becomes a meditation, and flexibility becomes a gateway to resilience.

Enhancing Flexibility

The pursuit of flexibility through gentle mobility workouts reveals its necessity not in the grand gestures of athleticism but in the quiet moments of everyday life. It is within the reach of a high shelf, the bend to tie a shoe, where the dividends of such practice manifest. Flexibility, cultivated through consistent engagement with mobility exercises, extends the body's vocabulary of movement, allowing for fluidity and ease that diminish the risk of strains and sprains. This extension of the body's capabilities acts as a bulwark against the rigidity and loss of motion that time may bring, ensuring that each day can be met with a full range of movement and the freedom it entails.

Yoga and Pilates

Within the realms of yoga and Pilates, the body finds a field for enhancing flexibility and a ground for strengthening its core and improving its balance. With its ancient roots and diverse expressions, yoga offers a journey through postures that challenge and fortify the body's stability and flexibility, each posing a conversation between muscle and breath. Pilates, focusing on the core as the center of strength, aligns the body in a harmony of movement and resistance, crafting a foundation upon which all physical activity can build. Together, these disciplines offer a holistic approach to mobility, where the benefits extend beyond the physical to touch upon the mental and emotional, fostering a well-being that is comprehensive and profound.

Routine Integration

The weaving of gentle mobility exercises into the fabric of one's weekly routine requires an intentionality that mirrors the deliberate nature of the movements themselves. It suggests a cadence where each day is met with a dedication to the movement, through the morning greeting with a series of yoga poses or the closure of the day with Pilates. This integration privileges consistency, recognizing that the actual value of these practices lies in their regular engagement, where the cumulative effect of daily dedication yields flexibility and strength that is both felt and seen. It is a commitment that fits not around one's life but seamlessly within it, a series of practices that become as natural and necessary as breathing.

Mind-Body Connection

The exploration of gentle mobility workouts reveals an aspect that transcends the physical, touching upon the mental and emotional realms where stress and tension often reside. The practice of yoga and Pilates, with their emphasis on mindful movement and breath, invites mindfulness that counterbalances the stresses of daily life. This mindfulness, cultivated on the mat, extends its serenity into the day, offering resilience against possible challenges. The connection between mind and body, forged through the repetition of these mobility exercises, becomes a source of strength and calm, where awareness of breath and movement serves as a reminder of the present moment's potential for peace and clarity.

In this dedicated exploration of gentle mobility workouts and their myriad benefits, from the enhancement of flexibility to the cultivation of a profound mind-body connection, one discovers a practice that is as nurturing as it is strengthening. The movements, though gentle, carry a potency that transcends their simplicity, offering a path to physical well-being that is balanced and holistic. Through the disciplines of yoga and Pilates, integrated thoughtfully into one's routine, the body finds mobility and resilience that support not just the physical demands of life but the emotional and mental as well, crafting wellness that is comprehensive, enduring, and deeply rooted in the harmonious dance of movement and stillness.

INTEGRATING EXERCISE INTO YOUR FASTING SCHEDULE

Marrying the rigors of intermittent fasting with the demands of physical activity necessitates a ballet of precision, where timing becomes a factor and a linchpin in optimizing energy utilization and recovery. This delicate orchestration, far from a rigid imposition, unfolds as a fluid dance, responsive to the body's rhythms and the nuances of individual metabolism. Within this interplay, discerning the optimal moments for exercise about fasting and feeding windows emerges as a critical skill, one honed through attentiveness to the body's feedback and the willingness to adapt.

Timing Matters

In this context, the clock serves as both a guide and an advisor, its hands pointing to opportunities where the body's readiness for exertion aligns with the nutritional support necessary for performance and recovery. For many, exercising toward the end of a fasting period harnesses a twofold advantage: firstly, engaging in physical activity when the body is primed to tap into fat reserves for energy, and secondly, positioning the subsequent feeding window as a prime time for nutrient absorption and recovery. This strategic placement ensures that the body, having expended its energy in the crucible of exercise, is met with the building blocks of repair and growth when it is most receptive.

Fasted Workouts

While inviting in theory, the concept of fasted workouts demands a nuanced approach in practice. At its core lies the potential for enhanced fat utilization. In this process, without readily available glucose from recent meals, the body turns to stored fat as its primary energy source. This shift, catalyzed by the hormonal landscape of fasting, particularly the rise in norepinephrine, suggests a metabolic efficiency that dovetails with the goals of many engaged in intermittent fasting. However, the effectiveness of fasted workouts is not universal but contingent on the individual's metabolic flexibility, the nature of the exercise, and the duration of the fasting period. It invites a dialogue with one's body. This listening discerns between the empowerment of fat utilization and the cautionary tale of potential muscle catabolism or undue fatigue.

Post-Workout Nutrition

Following the exertions of physical activity, especially within the crucible of fasting, the body stands at a crossroads, poised between the catabolic state induced by exercise and the anabolic potential of recovery. Post-workout nutrition emerges as a cornerstone, bridging the gap between depletion and replenishment. The immediacy and composition of this nutritional intervention are pivotal, with the post-exercise window—often pegged at the golden hour immediately following exertion—serving as a critical period for the absorption of carbohydrates and proteins. These nutrients, ingested in the aftermath of physical activity, act as the raw materials for the repair of muscle fibers and the replenishment of glycogen stores, ensuring that recovery is initiated and optimized. This approach underscores the importance of aligning the feeding window with exercise, ensuring that the body is not left wanting in the wake of its efforts.

Listening to Your Body

At the heart of integrating exercise into a fasting schedule lies a principle that transcends schedules, nutrient timing, and workout modalities: the imperative of listening to one's body. This attentiveness, an ongoing dialogue with the self, demands an openness to the signals of fatigue, hunger, and satiety, along with the subtler cues of mood and energy levels. It acknowledges that the body's needs fluctuate, influenced by the rhythm of fasting, the demands of exercise, and the stresses of daily life. Adjusting exercise intensity and duration in response to these cues becomes a practice of self-awareness, where the body's feedback shapes the approach to both fasting and physical activity. It is a dynamic process that eschews rigidity in favor of a responsiveness that honors the body's wisdom, ensuring that the marriage of intermittent fasting and exercise supports physical health and holistic well-being.

TRACKING FITNESS PROGRESS ALONGSIDE DIETARY CHANGES

In the quiet luminescence of dawn, when the world whispers promises of new beginnings, setting measurable fitness goals stands as a declaration, a testament to the will that propels one forward in the quest for health. This setting of goals, far from mere aspirations cast into the void, becomes a compass, guiding through the mists of uncertainty and the storms of doubt. These objectives, articulated with clarity and precision, span the breadth of physical endeavors, from the fortification of muscle to the enhancement of endurance, each a milestone in the odyssey of self-transformation. Beyond the simplistic measure of weight loss, these goals paint a portrait of health in broad strokes, capturing the nuances of vitality in their embrace.

The digital age, with its myriad innovations, offers tools of unparalleled sophistication for monitoring the progress that marches in lockstep with these ambitions. Fitness trackers and applications, the progeny of technology's union with wellness, serve as vigilant sentinels, recording each step taken, each heartbeat, and each moment of rest and exertion. This data, once the sole dominion of intuition, now finds form in graphs and numbers, a tangible record of the journey traversed. Adopting such technology, melding the human and the digital, allows for an introspection once deemed the realm of fantasy. Through these devices, the daily rituals of movement and the rhythms of rest unveil patterns, shedding light on the path toward the goals set with hopeful determination.

Reflection, a practice as ancient as humanity itself, finds new relevance in the context of this pursuit. In moments of solitude, when the world's clamor fades into the background, reflecting on the improvements witnessed becomes a source of sustenance. This contemplation, a mindful review of the strides made in strength, the bounds achieved in endurance, and the overall enhancement of fitness, feeds the flames of motivation. In these moments, the milestones, once distant, shimmer on the horizon with the promise of attainment. Personal and profound reflections remind one of the journey's worth, a narrative of progress that propels one forward, ever closer to the goals that beckon with the allure of fulfillment.

Integrating feedback, the fruit of this reflective practice, into the tapestry of exercise and dietary plans becomes an act of alchemy. The insights gleaned from the meticulous tracking of activity, the patterns unveiled through the application of technology, inform adjustments with the precision of a sculptor chiseling marble. This feedback, rich with personal experience data, illuminates the adjustments necessary for the diet and exercise regimen to evolve, ensuring that each step taken is one of informed confidence. Once guided by the nebulous dictates of tradition or convenience, dietary choices now focus on the clarity of personal health metrics. Similarly, the regimen of physical activity, informed by concrete evidence of progress, adapts, refining its focus to target areas of need with surgical precision.

In this meticulous orchestration of goals, tracking, reflection, and integration, the pursuit of health transcends the realm of the physical, touching the essence of personal transformation. The objectives outlined in the quiet of contemplation, pursued with the aid of technology and reflected upon with the wisdom of experience, chart a course through the uncharted waters of self-improvement. The feedback, a beacon in the night, guides the adjustments that ensure this course remains valid, a journey not just toward physical vitality but toward realizing one's fullest potential.

A harmony emerges in the interplay of light and shadow that dances across the landscape of health and wellness, the integration of exercise into the fabric of life, and the mindful adjustment of dietary habits in response to the body's dialogue. This harmony—a balance between the needs of the body and the aspirations of the spirit—becomes the foundation upon which the edifice of health is built.

CELEBRATING PHYSICAL ACHIEVEMENTS

In the realm of physical accomplishments, acknowledgment serves as the rich soil from which the seeds of motivation and satisfaction sprout. Recognizing milestones—those markers of progress that dot the landscape of our commitment to fitness—imbues the endeavor with meaning, transforming the abstract into the tangible. In this act of celebration, the essence of achievement finds its voice, a declaration that each step taken, each boundary pushed, enriches the narrative of personal growth.

Recognizing Milestones

The milestones punctuating the path of physical fitness, from the inaugural completion of a set distance to the triumphant mastery of a challenging yoga pose, demand acknowledgment. This recognition, reflective of the dedication and perseverance invested, acts as a mirror, reflecting the strength and resolve that characterize the pursuit of health. Acknowledging these milestones does more than mark progress; it reaffirms the commitment to oneself, a reminder that each step forward is a victory in its own right. Through this lens, milestones become not just markers of distance traveled but beacons of encouragement, illuminating the path ahead with the promise of potential yet to be realized.

Non-Scale Victories

In the shadow of the omnipresent scale, non-scale victories emerge as the unsung heroes of the fitness narrative. These triumphs, often unnoticed in pursuing numerical validation, carry an accurate measure of progress. The ability to climb stairs without pause, the newfound ease in bending and stretching, and the quiet retirement of once snug clothing—all speak to a transformation that numbers alone cannot capture. Focusing on these victories offers a broader perspective on health, encompassing strength, endurance, flexibility, and well-being beyond the confines of weight. In these achievements, the essence of actual progress is found, a testament to the holistic benefits of a committed fitness regimen.

Sharing Success

In sharing achievements with one's community, whether through social platforms, in the companionship of workout partners, or within the supportive embrace of a fitness class, a shared energy vibrates. This communal celebration acts as a catalyst, inspiring both the sharer and the audience, and is a reciprocal exchange of motivation and support. Sharing transcends mere narration, creating a tapestry of interconnected stories that are inspiring and uplifting. It fosters a sense of belonging, a recognition that the journey, while personal, is also shared—a collective endeavor buoyed by the successes of its members.

Rewarding Yourself

The reward, a concept as ancient as human endeavor itself, finds new expression in the context of physical achievements. Rewarding oneself for milestones reached or challenges overcome becomes a practice of positive reinforcement, a tangible acknowledgment of effort and perseverance. These rewards, chosen with care, reinforce healthy behaviors, serving as incentives that align with overall wellness goals. A massage to soothe tired muscles, a quiet afternoon with a beloved book, a particular class to refine a skill—all serve as rewards that nourish the body and the spirit, incentives that celebrate accomplishment while nurturing well-being. In this practice, the reward becomes a loop of positive feedback, each accomplishment celebrated and each celebration fostering further accomplishments.

In the constellation of physical fitness, where stars of achievements large and small dot the vastness of effort and dedication, celebration emerges as a fundamental force. Recognizing milestones, honoring non-scale victories, sharing successes, and rewarding oneself serve as a thread in the fabric of motivation, woven into a tapestry rich with personal meaning and communal inspiration. This fabric, resilient and vibrant, supports the ongoing commitment to health and well-being, a reminder that each step taken, each goal achieved, enriches not just the individual but the collective narrative of perseverance, strength, and growth.

As we draw the curtains on this exploration of physical achievements and their celebration, we are reminded of the intricate dance between individual effort and communal support, personal goals, and shared journeys. This dance, enriched by the recognition and celebration of each step forward, underscores the transformative power of fitness. This power extends beyond the physical to touch the very essence of well-being. It invites us to continue, to reach further, to climb higher, not just in pursuit of the next milestone but in the continuous exploration of our potential, a journey that unfolds with each breath, each movement, and each moment of celebration.

MENTAL AND EMOTIONAL WELL-BEING – THE FASTING MIND

In the quiet before dawn, when the world holds its breath, awaiting the first light, there's a space where silence speaks volumes. It's in this space that the mind finds its serenity, a pause between yesterday's cacophony and today's demands. Intermittent fasting, often perceived through the lens of physical health, extends its influence far beyond touching mental clarity and emotional balance. This chapter navigates the nuanced topography of the mind under the gentle discipline of fasting, revealing a landscape where cognitive fog clears, and emotional tumult finds its calm.

THE IMPACT OF FASTING ON MENTAL CLARITY AND MOOD

Brain Health Benefits

The brain, that intricate orchestrator of thought, emotion, and memory, thrives under the watchful care of intermittent fasting.

By moderating blood sugar levels and reducing inflammation, this practice lays the groundwork for enhanced cognitive function. It's akin to decluttering a once crowded room, where each removed item—a spike in glucose here, a swell of inflammation there—adds to the clarity and functionality of the space. The result is a mind unburdened, capable of higher thought processes, improved focus, and agility in problem-solving that was once obscured by the haze of dietary excess.

Consider, for instance, the simple act of organizing a library. As books are sorted and shelves cleared, finding a desired volume becomes less frustrating and more seamless. Similarly, fasting helps streamline the body's metabolic processes, affording the brain clarity that enhances our ability to navigate complex tasks and challenges with ease.

Mood Regulation

Fasting's influence extends into emotional health, stabilizing the often tumultuous seas of mood fluctuations. By impacting the regulation of neurotransmitters such as serotonin and dopamine, fasting can mitigate the sharp edges of anxiety and soften the depths of depression. This effect is not unlike the calm that follows a storm, where the air, once heavy with tension, clears to reveal a sky of tranquil blue. The practice of fasting, in moderating the body's hormonal responses, acts as a balm, soothing the frayed edges of our emotional tapestries.

Nutritional Support for the Brain

During fasting periods, emphasizing nutrient-dense foods within eating windows becomes a cornerstone of cognitive and emotional health. In particular, omega-3 fatty acids, antioxidants, and B vitamins play pivotal roles in supporting brain function and mood regulation. Imagine crafting a meal as one would compose a symphony, where each nutrient adds a note to the harmony of mental well-being. The strategic inclusion of foods rich in these nutrients during eating windows nourishes the body. It fortifies the mind against the rigors of stress and the wear of time.

Personal Testimonials

The narratives of those who have woven intermittent fasting into their lives speak volumes of its impact on mental and emotional well-being. In forums, blogs, and discussions, individuals recount experiences of heightened clarity, a newfound calm in the face of stress, and a joy in the simplicity of living that was once muted by constant dietary indulgence. These stories, each unique in its contours, share a common thread—a testament to the transformative power of fasting on the mind and spirit.

Textual Element: A Fasting Mind Checklist

To navigate the mental and emotional landscape of intermittent fasting, consider the following:

- Daily Reflections: Dedicate a few moments each day to reflect on changes in mood and mental clarity. Note improvements or challenges.
- Nutrient Log: Track your intake of brain-supportive nutrients during eating windows. Aim for a balanced intake of omega-3s, antioxidants, and B vitamins.
- Mood Monitor: Keep a simple log of mood fluctuations. Over time, look for patterns that may correlate with fasting periods or specific foods.

- Community Connection: Engage with online forums or local groups to share experiences and strategies for supporting mental well-being through fasting.

In the unfolding narrative of intermittent fasting, the chapters dedicated to physical health are richly complemented by the sections exploring mental and emotional well-being. The mind, once clouded by the fog of nutritional excess, finds in fasting a path to clarity and calm—a journey not of deprivation but of discovery. As the body adapts to the rhythms of fasting and feeding, so does the spirit, embracing a simplicity that brings focus to the present and hope to the future. Between the silence of fasting and the abundance of feeding lies the potential for a well-being that encompasses the totality of the human experience, inviting us to explore the depths of our minds and the breadth of our emotional landscapes with newfound clarity and peace.

STRESS MANAGEMENT TECHNIQUES FOR SUSTAINABLE FASTING

In the realm where silence meets the cacophony of life's relentless pace, stress carves its indelible marks, subtly influencing the ebb and flow of our fasting endeavors and the broader canvas of our health. The intricate dance of managing these stressors demands a choreography that respects the delicate balance between action and repose, between the stirring of ambition and the solace of tranquility. In this fragile equilibrium, identifying and managing stressors emerges not as a mere strategy but as a vital necessity, ensuring that our fasting practices and overall well-being remain unscathed by the tumultuous undercurrents of daily life.

Identifying stressors requires an introspection that pierces through the superficial layers of discomfort to reveal the root causes that disturb our peace. This process, akin to tracing the source of a river back to its hidden spring, demands patience and a willingness to confront truths that may lie buried beneath the debris of denial and distraction. As we map these stressors, from the pressures of professional commitments to the whispers of unresolved personal conflicts, we arm ourselves with the knowledge necessary to navigate through the storms they conjure.

The arsenal against stress is ancient and ever-evolving, a testament to humanity's quest for equilibrium. Among these tools, relaxation techniques are pillars of resilience, offering refuge and restoration. With its roots entwined with the earliest human civilizations, meditation beckons us into a realm of stillness, where the mind, untethered from the constant demands of thought, finds a sanctuary in the present. This simple yet profound practice aligns the rhythms of breath with the cadence of tranquility, weaving a tapestry of peace that shields the spirit from the assaults of anxiety and unrest.

Deep breathing, an act as instinctive as it is overlooked, offers a bridge to calm, a method by which the storm of stress is quelled through the deliberate modulation of breath. Each inhalation, deep and unhurried, carries the promise of oxygen-rich clarity. At the same time, every exhalation bears away the remnants of tension, a cycle of renewal that roots us firmly in the realm of serenity. Mindfulness, a companion to meditation, invites us to live fully, embracing each moment with an attentiveness that transforms mundane acts into awareness rituals. In this heightened state of consciousness, stress is not so much eradicated as it is transcended, its edges softened by the gentle embrace of acceptance and presence.

Balancing lifestyle factors, a task as demanding as it is rewarding, requires an orchestration that honors the rhythms of both work and rest. In pursuing this balance, the boundaries between professional endeavors and personal respite must be delineated with care, ensuring that the sanctuary of leisure remains intact against the encroachments of work. This distinction, while firm, allows for a fluidity that accommodates the unpredictability of life. This flexibility embraces the necessity of rest as fervently as it champions the virtues of labor. In this equilibrium, fasting finds fertile ground, supported by a lifestyle that nurtures both the body and the mind.

Yet, there are moments when the weight of stress fractures even the sturdiest of defenses, moments when the guidance of professionals becomes not just a resource but a lifeline. In these instances, seeking support is an act of courage, a recognition that the path to well-being sometimes requires the companionship of those skilled in navigating the mazes of the mind. Therapists, counselors, and mentors offer their expertise as a beacon, illuminating the steps toward healing and equilibrium. This partnership, rooted in trust and mutual respect, forges a bridge over the chasms of stress, leading us toward a terrain where fasting and health flourish, unburdened by the shadows of distress.

In the tapestry of our lives, where threads of joy are interwoven with strands of challenge, stress management stands as a skill honed through identification, relaxation, lifestyle balance, and the seeking of supportive guidance. Each technique, each strategy we employ, adds a layer of resilience to our being, a fortification against the vicissitudes of existence. As we navigate through the intricacies of fasting, mindful of the stresses that buffet our journey, we cultivate a strength that sustains us, a serenity that guides us, and a well-being that defines us, unfettered by the tumult that life may bring.

BUILDING A SUPPORTIVE COMMUNITY

In the tapestry of human experience, the threads of connection and camaraderie weave patterns of support and solidarity, crafting a fabric that envelopes us in times of need and celebration. The adoption of intermittent fasting, a path marked by its own set of challenges and triumphs, calls for the warmth of this fabric, inviting the formation of a community where shared experiences and mutual understanding foster a sense of belonging. This network, formed of like-minded individuals, emerges not as a luxury but as a necessity, providing a foundation upon which the edifice of personal transformation can securely rest.

Finding Like-Minded Individuals

The quest for companions who share a commitment to intermittent fasting begins with a step into the vast garden of human connection, where the seeds of friendship and camaraderie await their moment to bloom. This search, guided by intention and curiosity, finds its roots in the common ground of shared goals and experiences. Engaging in conversations at health seminars, participating in wellness workshops, or simply sharing one's fasting story can attract those on a similar path, drawing them closer like moths to a flame. These initial interactions, tentative yet tinged with the promise of understanding, lay the groundwork for relationships that can withstand the ebbs and flows of personal health journeys.

Online and Local Groups

In the digital age, the quest for community transcends the limitations of geography, reaching into the virtual realm where forums and social media groups abound. These platforms, pulsating with the lifeblood of shared interests, offer a sanctuary for those seeking advice, encouragement, and the simple recognition of their efforts. Similarly, local health clubs and community centers often host groups dedicated to fasting and wellness, providing a space where the tangible presence of others adds weight to words of support. In the confluence of online and offline gatherings, community bonds are forged and strengthened by the shared pursuit of health and well-being.

The Role of Community in Motivation

Within the embrace of a supportive community, motivation finds fertile soil nurtured by its members' collective energy and aspirations. The tales of triumph and the honest admissions of setbacks shared among peers act as both a mirror and a beacon, reflecting our struggles and illuminating the path ahead. The encouragement received in moments of doubt, and the shared joy in each milestone reached serve as reminders of the strength that lies in unity. This communal motivation, a force more potent than any individual resolve, becomes an inexhaustible wellspring from which we can draw during moments of faltering will.

Creating Your Support System

The architecture of a support system, tailored to the intricacies of one's fasting journey, requires a discerning eye and an open heart. Begin by identifying those in your immediate circle who express genuine interest in and understanding of your goals. Whether they partake in fasting or not, these individuals become the cornerstone of your support, offering a listening ear and a shoulder to lean on. Expanding this nucleus to include fasting peers and mentors adds expertise and empathy, creating a multidimensional network encompassing a wide range of experiences and insights.

Engaging family and friends in meal planning and preparation can transform fasting from a solitary endeavor into a shared activity, imbuing it with a sense of communal purpose. This inclusivity not only demystifies the process for loved ones but also integrates fasting into the fabric of daily life, making it a shared narrative rather than an individual subplot. Additionally, initiating or joining fasting challenges within your community can catalyze a collective momentum, turning the pursuit of health into a shared adventure marked by camaraderie and collective achievement.

In constructing this support system, consider the creation of a fasting circle, a dedicated group that meets regularly to share meals, discuss challenges, and celebrate successes. This circle, bound by the common threads of fasting and friendship, becomes a microcosm of the larger community, providing a space where intimacy and understanding deepen the roots of support. Through social media or local community boards, reach out to those who might share your commitment to fasting and wellness, inviting them to join in creating a collective that thrives on mutual support and shared goals.

As this network of support takes shape, weaving its way through the landscape of your fasting journey, remember that its strength lies not just in the advice or encouragement received but in the profound sense of belonging it fosters. This community, built on the foundation of shared experience and mutual respect, becomes a haven where the challenges of fasting are met with under-standing and compassion, where triumphs are celebrated with genuine joy, and where the journey toward health and well-being is a passage walked together, each step buoyed by the strength of collective resolve and the warmth of human connection.

CULTIVATING A POSITIVE MINDSET TOWARD AGING

In the quiet theater of our later years, where shadows lengthen, and the play of life takes on a richer hue, the narrative of aging undergoes a profound transformation. This period, often portrayed through a lens of decline, holds within its folds a potential for renewal and growth that challenges the foundations of societal preconceptions. It invites a reevaluation of aging, not as a diminution of self but as an expansion, where the accumulation of years brings a depth of wisdom, a resilience of spirit, and a beauty that defies the superficial judgments of youth.

The act of challenging age stereotypes begins with a dismantling of the myths that shroud our later years in apprehension and misconceptions. It confronts the narrative of inevitable decline with evidence of vitality, creativity, and ongoing growth that characterizes so many lives well beyond the arbitrary milestones of middle age. This confrontation is not a denial of the physical changes accompanying aging but an affirmation of the countless ways individuals continue to evolve, contribute, and flourish. It draws upon the myriad examples of those who, in the twilight of their years, embark on new ventures, master new skills, and discover new passions, illustrating that the potential for achievement and fulfillment knows no age limit.

Celebrating age and experience becomes an act of defiance against a culture that too often equates worth with youth and overlooks the beauty inherent in accumulating life's moments. This celebration acknowledges the lines etched by laughter and sorrow as badges of honor, testaments to a life of intensity and purpose. It sees in the graying hair and the softened contours of the body a map of journeys undertaken, challenges met, and loves embraced. This perspective elevates aging from a process of loss to one of gain, where every year adds to the richness of our character and the depth of our understanding.

The link between a positive mindset and increased longevity and quality of life is not merely anecdotal but grounded in a growing body of scientific evidence. Studies reveal that those who view aging with optimism and a sense of purpose are likelier to experience better health outcomes, lower stress levels, and greater satisfaction with life. This correlation underscores the power of mindset in navigating the waters of aging, suggesting that the stories we tell ourselves about what it means to grow older can shape our reality. It posits that by cultivating an attitude of gratitude, resilience, and openness to the unfolding adventure of life, we can not only enhance our well-being but also serve as beacons for others as they navigate their paths through the later years.

Inspirational stories of individuals who have embraced aging with grace and vigor illuminate the possibilities that await us. Consider the artist who finds her most authentic voice in the quiet of retirement, her canvases a riot of color and emotion that draw acclaim from far and wide. Or the athlete who, at an age when many have long since retreated from the arena of competition, trains with the dedication of a novice, his sights set on marathons yet to be run. These stories, each unique in their trajectory, share a common theme: a refusal to be defined by the number of years lived and a determination to explore, grow, and contribute.

These narratives, drawn from the lives of those around us and the annals of history, serve as sources of inspiration and reminders of our potential. They invite us to look beyond the societal scripts that too often dictate what aging should look like and encourage us to author our stories of vitality, creativity, and continual growth. In their triumphs and challenges, we find reflections of our possibilities, a mirror that reveals not the limitations of age but the boundless horizon that lies before us.

In this reimagining of aging, where stereotypes are challenged, experiences celebrated, and the link between mindset and longevity embraced, we find a landscape rich with potential. It is a realm where the wisdom gleaned from years lived is the currency of true wealth, where the resilience born of navigating life's trials becomes a wellspring of strength, and where the beauty of aging is acknowledged in the depth of character, the warmth of relationships, and the vibrancy of ongoing endeavors. This perspective on aging, rooted in positivity and bolstered by the inspirational stories of those who tread this path with courage and joy, offers a blueprint for a life not diminished by the passage of time but enriched by it. In this life, every moment is an opportunity for growth, connection, and the celebration of the enduring spirit.

OVERCOMING PLATEAUS AND STAYING MOTIVATED

In the intricate dance of intermittent fasting, there comes a moment, often unexpected yet inevitably encountered, where the rhythm falters, steps once lively and assured now tread in place. This plateau, a landscape seemingly devoid of progression, presents itself not as an insurmountable barrier but as an inherent aspect of the fasting voyage. Within these stretches of apparent stasis, the body, in its wisdom, pauses, recalibrating and consolidating gains beneath the surface, unseen yet profoundly transformative. Recognizing these plateaus for what they genuinely signify —a natural recalibration rather than a cessation of progress— shifts the perception, illuminating them as waypoints rather than termini.

The metaphorical toolbox for navigating these plateaus brims with strategies; each instrument is honed for reigniting momentum.

The first and most potent tool involves recalibrating one's fasting regimen. Introducing variability, whether through adjusting the duration of fasting windows or experimenting with different fasting protocols, injects a dynamic element into the routine. This variability, akin to altering the course of a river, revitalizes the metabolic processes, encouraging the body to adapt anew. It mirrors introducing a novel species into a garden, where the new entrant stimulates growth and vitality, enriching the ecosystem.

Parallel to this physiological recalibration, the nurturing of motivation becomes paramount. Here, the setting of micro-goals, achievable and succinct objectives, offers a series of attainable victories, each small win a kindle for the flame of motivation. This segmentation of larger ambitions into a mosaic of micro-goals transforms an overwhelming landscape into a series of manageable steps, each victory a testament to persistence. It's akin to the meticulous assembly of a mosaic, where each tiny, colored piece contributes to the emergence of a vibrant, cohesive whole, the beauty of the final image rendered all the more exquisite by the intricacy of its composition.

In this odyssey, adjusting expectations emerges as a guiding star. It demands a shift in perspective, where success is measured not solely by the milestones of weight loss or fitness achievements but by the richness of the experience and the depth of personal growth. This recalibration of expectations fosters kindness toward oneself, an acknowledgment that the value of the fasting journey lies as much in the lessons learned and the resilience built as in the tangible outcomes. It mirrors cultivating a garden, where the true reward lies in the harvest and the quiet satisfaction of tending and nurturing, of witnessing growth and change.

Cultivating motivation in the face of plateaus also draws upon the power of reflection and celebration. In moments of stillness, reflecting on the distance traversed, the challenges surmounted, and the growth attained offers a wellspring of motivation. This reflection, a deliberate pause to honor the journey thus far, reminds one of one's capability and strength. Celebrating not just the milestones but also the effort expended and the perseverance shown becomes an act of self-recognition, a recognition that bolsters the spirit and renews the commitment to the path chosen. It is akin to pausing on a trek to look back upon the path climbed, where the perspective gained from the vantage point offers a sense of accomplishment and a renewed vigor to continue the ascent.

The journey through intermittent fasting, marked by its peaks and valleys, its moments of swift progress, and stretches of stillness, mirrors the broader voyage of life. In the embrace of plateaus, the recalibration of strategies, the nurturing of motivation, the adjustment of expectations, and the celebration of both victories and efforts lie a microcosm of living. Each plateau is overcome, each motivation is sustained, each expectation is adjusted, and each achievement is celebrated, enriching the tapestry of the fasting experience and weaving resilience, growth, and satisfaction into its fabric. With its inherent challenges and rewards, this journey becomes not just a pathway to physical health but a profound exploration of the self, a testament to the indomitable spirit that propels us forward, ever onward, through the ever-changing landscape of life.

ADDRESSING SOCIAL ISOLATION THROUGH SHARED MEAL PLANNING

Navigating the intricacies of social engagements while steadfastly adhering to an intermittent fasting schedule emerges as a delicate challenge. The friendliness of shared meals, a cornerstone of human interaction, often finds itself at odds with the disciplined structure of fasting. This divergence need not predicate a retreat into isolation; instead, it beckons a creative reimagining of communal dining that honors the spirit of togetherness and the sanctity of one's fasting regimen.

The endeavor of shared meal planning unfurls as a tapestry woven with threads of compromise, understanding, and mutual respect. It begins with an open dialogue, an invitation extended to friends and family to partake in crafting a meal experience that transcends dietary constraints. This collaborative effort, rooted in the desire for inclusivity, transforms meal planning from a solitary task into a collective journey. It is akin to orchestrating a symphony where each participant contributes a unique melody, resulting in a harmonious blend that resonates with shared satisfaction.

In this collaborative space, the conception of fasting-friendly gatherings takes shape, embodying a fusion of creativity and flexibility. Brunches timed to coincide with the closing of one's fasting window or dinners scheduled within the golden hours of nutritional replenishment offer a canvas upon which diverse culinary preferences can coalesce. These gatherings, characterized by their adaptability, serve not as reminders of dietary divergence but as celebrations of shared moments. They testify that the heart of social dining beats not in the specifics of what is consumed but in the joy of companionship and the warmth of shared experiences.

The articulation of dietary needs, a task often fraught with apprehension, unfolds gracefully when approached with positivity and assurance. It is less a declaration of restrictions than an invitation to explore the vast expanse of culinary possibilities within the framework of intermittent fasting. Communicating these needs, therefore, becomes an exercise in diplomacy, one that educates and enlightens, dispelling misconceptions and fostering an environment of support and understanding. It is through this transparent exchange that misconceptions are dismantled, and the path to enjoyable, inclusive dining experiences is laid bare.

Adopting these strategies recedes the specter of social isolation, revealing a landscape where fasting and fellowship flourish in tandem. It is a landscape marked by meals that nourish both body and soul, where laughter and conversation flow as freely as the dishes that grace the table. This approach to social dining, characterized by its inclusivity and creativity, reinforces that intermittent fasting, far from a solitary endeavor, is enriched by the company we keep and the meals we share.

In reflection, the journey through shared meal planning and fasting-friendly gatherings illuminates a path where the challenges of social eating are met with innovative solutions. It underscores the power of communication in bridging dietary divides. It highlights the importance of creativity in redefining the boundaries of communal dining. This journey, woven into the broader narrative of intermittent fasting, serves as a reminder that the quest for health and well-being is not a road traveled alone but a voyage enriched by the presence of others. It affirms that within the tapestry of human connection lies strength and resilience that nourish us, body and soul, guiding us forward into the chapters yet to unfold.

BEYOND THE BASICS –
ELEVATING AUTOPHAGY FOR
LONGEVITY

In the serene predawn, where the only sound is the gentle rustle of leaves in the soft morning breeze, a profound transformation occurs not in the world around us but within the cells that constitute our being. This silent metamorphosis, known as autophagy, is the body's way of cleansing itself of damaged components, ensuring the renewal and maintenance of cellular health. Imagine a scenario as commonplace as cleaning one's house. Just as we periodically clear away clutter and dust to maintain a healthy living environment, autophagy also tidies our cellular landscape, promoting longevity and vitality.

AUTOPHAGY AND ITS ROLE IN LONGEVITY

Cellular Renewal Mechanism

Autophagy, a term derived from the Greek words for "self" and "eating," is a process by which cells degrade and recycle their own components. This cellular housekeeping is crucial for removing dysfunctional proteins and organelles, akin to replacing old, worn-out machinery in a factory with new, efficient models. The result is a rejuvenated cellular environment conducive to optimal function and resilience against stressors.

Triggering Autophagy

Intermittent fasting emerges as a key activator of autophagy, initiating this cleansing process through periods of energy restriction. It's worth noting that the fasting duration required to trigger autophagy can vary, with research suggesting that extended periods of fasting—beyond the 16-hour mark—might be necessary to elicit significant autophagic activity. This activation is akin to rebooting a computer, where a temporary shutdown allows system optimization and clears unnecessary files, enhancing performance upon restart.

Autophagy and Aging

A robust body of scientific evidence underscores the pivotal role of autophagy in mitigating the aging process. Studies have illuminated how enhanced autophagy contributes to an extended lifespan in various organisms, from simple yeast to more complex mammals. This link between autophagy and aging posits that by maintaining cellular integrity and function, autophagy can decelerate aging, paving the way for a longer and healthier life. One can liken this to regular vehicle maintenance, where routine checks and repairs can significantly extend its operational lifespan while preventing a decline in performance.

Maximizing Autophagy Benefits

A strategic approach to the timing and frequency of fasting periods is essential to leveraging the full spectrum of autophagy's benefits through intermittent fasting. Incorporating longer fasts, such as 24-hour periods every few weeks, alongside daily shorter fasts, can create a conducive environment for autophagy, ensuring cells remain vigilant in their housekeeping duties. Moreover, complementing fasting with exercise and a diet rich in nutrients known to support autophagy, such as spermidine, can amplify the process further.

Visual Element: Autophagy Activation Timeline

A detailed infographic illustrates the autophagy activation and fasting duration timeline, providing a visual guide to optimizing one's fasting schedule for maximal autophagic benefit. This timeline, grounded in scientific research, demystifies the process. It offers readers a clear, actionable blueprint for integrating fasting into their routines to promote cellular health and longevity.

In the stillness of the morning, as the world awakens to the promise of a new day, our cells, too, awaken to the opportunity for renewal through autophagy. This silent yet profound process, catalyzed by intermittent fasting, holds the key to extending our lifespan and enhancing our life's quality. By embracing fasting as a trigger for autophagy, we unlock the door to cellular health, ensuring that each cell, like each day, is met with the vigor of renewal and the promise of vitality.

FASTING MIMICKING DIETS AND THEIR POTENTIAL

A nuanced approach to dietary sustenance, fasting mimicking diets (FMD) represents a confluence of tradition and innovation, simulating the physiological benefits of fasting while permitting food intake. This methodology, intricate in its design, orchestrates a dietary pattern that mirrors the metabolic and cellular effects of true fasting, offering a bridge for those for whom traditional fasting presents insurmountable challenges. At its core, FMD operates under a paradigm that reduces caloric intake significantly for a set duration, typically five consecutive days, thereby coaxing the body into a state that echoes the fasting experience without complete abstention from food.

The genesis of FMD lies in an endeavor to distill the essence of fasting's benefits into a form that enhances compliance and accessibility, thereby expanding the reach of fasting's health-promoting potential. This diet, meticulously structured to maintain nutritional balance while limiting caloric input, ignites a cascade of biological processes akin to those activated during traditional fasting periods. Among these, cellular rejuvenation stands out as prominent, a process in which the body, recognizing the simulated fast, initiates an internal overhaul, clearing away cellular detritus and refurbishing the machinery of life at the molecular level.

The implications of FMD for metabolic health unfold in a tapestry of improved biomarkers, including but not limited to enhanced glucose regulation, reduced inflammation, and a favorable shift in lipid profiles. These alterations in the body's biochemical milieu contribute to a fortified defense against the onset of aging-associated diseases, casting FMD as a beacon for those navigating the complexities of metabolic syndromes and other chronic conditions. The diet's capacity to modulate risk factors associated with cardiovascular diseases, diabetes, and neurodegenerative disorders positions it as a compelling adjunct to lifestyle interventions aimed at disease prevention and health span extension.

Implementing an FMD necessitates a thoughtful curation of meals, where macronutrient composition and caloric content are calibrated to mimic the fasting state without crossing the threshold into nutritional deprivation. The diet's typically plant-based architecture leans heavily on nutrient-dense foods that deliver high satiety and ample micronutrients at a reduced caloric load. This orchestration of dietary elements requires diligent planning, ensuring that each meal, though modest in energy contribution, serves as a vessel for essential vitamins, minerals, and phytonutrients. Including foods rich in healthy fats, such as avocados and nuts, alongside ample vegetables and legumes, crafts a dietary scaffold that supports the body's needs during this simulated fast, ensuring that nutritional integrity is preserved even as caloric intake is curtailed.

Recent explorations into the efficacy of FMD shed light on its potential as a revolutionary approach to health maintenance and disease mitigation. Emerging studies underscore the diet's impact on biomarkers of longevity, with evidence pointing to the activation of pathways associated with lifespan extension, metabolic health, and cognitive function. These investigations, rigorous in their methodology, offer a glimpse into the transformative potential of FMD, suggesting that the benefits traditionally ascribed to prolonged fasting may be attainable through this more accessible and manageable dietary strategy.

As the landscape of nutritional science evolves, the fasting-mimicking diet stands at the vanguard, challenging conventional fasting and food restriction paradigms. It extends an invitation to those who seek the profound benefits of fasting but are deterred by the prospect of complete food abstention, offering a meticulously crafted alternative that promises rejuvenation, health, and vitality. In this light, FMD emerges not merely as a dietary regimen but as a testament to the ingenuity of human endeavor to harness the ancient wisdom of fasting, reimagined for the modern age.

THE SCIENCE OF SLEEP AND FASTING

In the still tapestry of night, when the world surrenders to rest, profound alchemy occurs within the confines of our body, a transformation where the realms of sleep and fasting intertwine in a delicate ballet. This interplay, marked by a complexity that defies simple explanation, is key to unlocking a state of well-being that extends its influence far beyond waking hours, seeping into the very fabric of our existence.

Interconnectedness of Sleep and Fasting

The intricate relationship between sleep quality and fasting emerges from the depths of our biological rhythms, where circadian clocks orchestrate the symphony of our bodily functions. Fasting, in its disciplined abstention from nourishment, exerts a subtle yet significant impact on these rhythms, nudging the pendulum of our internal clocks toward a harmony that resonates with our natural sleep cycles. Conversely, the embrace of sleep, with its restorative phases of deep slumber and REM cycles, influences the efficacy of fasting, setting the stage for a cycle of renewal that is both nourished and nurtured by rest.

Improving Sleep through Fasting

The promise of fasting as a harbinger of enhanced sleep quality unfolds within the embrace of night, where the cessation of digestion allows the body to turn its focus inward, channeling its energies toward repair and rejuvenation. This shift away from the metabolic demands of digestion toward the restorative processes of sleep ushers in an improvement in both the depth and quality of slumber. The stages of REM and deep sleep—those bastions of mental and physical renewal—are bolstered by the fasting state, their benefits magnified in the absence of dietary distractions. In this landscape, the mind, unburdened by the task of processing the day's intake, ventures into realms of dreams and deep thought, emerging refreshed and invigorated at dawn's light.

Fasting and Hormones

The cascade of hormonal fluctuations accompanying the fasting state plays a pivotal role in the orchestration of sleep quality. Melatonin, the herald of sleep's onset, finds its production subtly influenced by the rhythms of fasting, its levels attuned to the ebb and flow of nourishment and abstention. Cortisol, the sentinel of wakefulness, observes a recalibration in response to fasting, its peaks and valleys aligning with the cycles of feeding and fasting, ensuring that its surge at dawn dovetails with our natural propensity to awaken. This dance of hormones, guided by the fasting state, fosters an environment conducive to sleep, where the body's chemical messengers align in support of restful slumber.

Sleep Strategies While Fasting

In navigating the nocturnal realms while engaged in fasting, a tapestry of strategies unfurls, each thread woven to enhance sleep quality. The timing of exercise, when aligned with the waning light of day, primes the body for rest, its exertions signaling the approach of night and the need for restoration. The final meal, curated to satiate without overburdening, sets the stage for a night of undisturbed sleep, its composition mindful of the delicate balance between nourishment and rest. Together, these strategies form a mosaic of practices that honor the sanctity of sleep in the fasting state, ensuring that each night's journey into slumber is met with ease and grace.

INTERMITTENT FASTING AND GUT HEALTH: A NEW FRONTIER

Gut Health Basics

In the labyrinth of the human body, the gut stands as a critical nexus. In this complex ecosystem, trillions of microorganisms— bacteria, viruses, and fungi—coexist in a delicate balance. This microbiome, which encapsulates this vast array of life, operates not in isolation but in profound symbiosis with its host, influencing a spectrum of physiological functions from nutrient absorption to immune system modulation. The equilibrium of this microbial community is a testament to the body's resilience, adapting to the ebb and flow of dietary patterns, environmental factors, and the rhythm of life itself. Understanding the foundational role of gut health necessitates an appreciation for this intricate dance of microorganisms, recognizing their influence on not just digestive efficiency but the overarching well-being of their human host.

Fasting and Microbiome Diversity

The introduction of intermittent fasting into this dynamic environment initiates a cascade of changes, subtle yet significant in their impact on the diversity and composition of the gut microbiome. This alteration in dietary rhythm, characterized by intervals of nourishment followed by periods of abstention, fosters an environment where specific microbial populations thrive. In contrast, others wane, a shift that mirrors the natural cycles of feast and famine. This oscillation in microbial abundance and diversity, far from a mere consequence of altered food intake, reflects a more profound adaptation to the fasting state, with potential implications for gut health and beyond. The enrichment of microbial species associated with enhanced metabolic regulation and reduced inflammation suggests a link between fasting, microbiome diversity, and the body's capacity for self-regulation and disease resistance.

Benefits for Digestive Health

The implications of intermittent fasting for digestive health unfold against the backdrop of this microbial reshaping, where reductions in inflammation and improvements in gut barrier function emerge as tangible benefits. By modulating the activity and composition of the gut microbiome, the fasting state may contribute to a reduction in the inflammatory signals that permeate the gut barrier, a phenomenon associated with a spectrum of digestive disorders. Concurrently, the reinforcement of the gut barrier, a critical defense against the incursion of harmful substances, underscores the potential of fasting to fortify the body's natural protection. This dual action, reducing inflammation while enhancing barrier integrity, encapsulates the promise of intermittent fasting as a modality for digestive health, offering a pathway to alleviate discomfort and mitigate the risk of chronic conditions rooted in gut dysfunction.

Personalizing Fasting for Gut Health

Navigating the realm of intermittent fasting to optimize gut health invites a personalized approach that considers the nuances of individual microbiomes and dietary preferences. The selection of foods within eating windows becomes a critical consideration, emphasizing those known to nourish the gut microbiome—fibrous vegetables, fermented foods, and polyphenol-rich fruits stand as pillars of a microbiome-friendly diet. This strategic nourishment, aligned with the timing and duration of fasting periods, allows for a tailored fasting experience that supports the growth of beneficial microbial populations while respecting the body's unique dietary needs. The integration of probiotic and prebiotic supplements, under the guidance of healthcare professionals, may further enhance this personalization, offering targeted support to the microbiome during periods of fasting.

Exploring intermittent fasting as a conduit for gut health enhancement marks a convergence of ancient practices with modern scientific understanding. This fusion promises a new frontier in the pursuit of well-being. This journey, grounded in the recognition of the gut microbiome's pivotal role in overall health, harnesses the transformative potential of fasting to reshape the digestive landscape.

ADVANCED TRACKING: BEYOND WEIGHT AND MEASUREMENTS

Holistic Health Tracking

In an era where the quantification of health often reduces it to mere numbers on a scale or the circumference of a waist, a more nuanced approach beckons, embracing a broad spectrum of biomarkers to illuminate the multifaceted landscape of well-being. This holistic tracking transcends traditional metrics, delving into the biochemical and physiological narratives that unfold beneath the surface, narratives that reveal the intricate interplay between fasting, metabolism, and cellular health. Here, in the aggregation of data points from blood glucose levels to markers of inflammation, a comprehensive portrait of health emerges, offering insights far more prosperous than those gleaned from physical measurements alone. This approach, meticulous in its attention to detail, affords precision in customizing fasting regimens, tailoring them to each individual's unique needs and goals.

Monitoring Metabolic Health

Monitoring metabolic health indicators, a practice both art and science, requires an attentiveness to the body's subtle cues, an attentiveness cultivated through the regular assessment of key biomarkers. Blood glucose levels, a mirror reflecting the body's capacity to manage sugar, offer a glimpse into the metabolic efficiency honed by fasting. Lipid profiles, with their tales of cholesterol and triglycerides, speak volumes about cardiovascular health and the risk of chronic disease. When tracked over time, these indicators chart the impact of fasting on metabolic function, guiding adjustments in dietary timing and composition to optimize health outcomes. It is a meticulous process, akin to tuning a fine instrument, where each adjustment brings the body closer to its optimal state of harmony.

Tracking Autophagy and Gut Health Indicators

Pursuing markers that signal the activation of autophagy and the state of gut health ventures into territories less charted but no less significant. The detection of autophagy, a process shrouded in cellular complexity, challenges the limits of current technology. Yet, emerging research offers promising avenues for its indirect assessment. Biomarkers such as levels of particular lipids or proteins associated with autophagic activity hint at the presence of this cellular renewal, providing a window into the fasting-induced rejuvenation occurring out of sight. Similarly, the composition of the gut microbiome, with its vast array of species, reflects the influence of fasting on digestive health. Advances in genomic sequencing allow for a detailed analysis of microbial diversity, offering a metric by which the benefits of fasting on gut health can be quantified. These indicators, though complex, pave the way for a deeper understanding of fasting's systemic effects, illuminating paths to enhanced well-being.

Utilizing Wearable Technology

Wearable technology has revolutionized health metrics tracking, transforming the abstract into the tangible and the invisible into the visible. Devices that monitor heart rate variability, sleep patterns, and activity levels now offer insights into the body's response to fasting, providing real-time feedback on the physiological shifts accompanying periods of abstention from food. This technology, sophisticated in its capabilities, allows for a nuanced analysis of fasting's effects, from the subtle changes in stress levels indicated by heart rate variability to the improvements in sleep quality captured by nocturnal monitoring. Integrating these devices into the fasting experience offers a data-rich narrative of health that informs and guides the optimization of fasting schedules for maximum benefit. It is a confluence of innovation and tradition, where the ancient practice of fasting meets the cutting edge of technology, each enhancing the other in the pursuit of health and vitality.

In the tapestry of health tracking, each thread represents a different biomarker or metric; a rich and detailed picture of well-being emerges, which defies reduction to simple measurements. This holistic approach, embracing the complexity and diversity of health indicators, offers a roadmap to personalized fasting regimens, each tailored to the nuanced needs of the individual. It is a journey informed by data, guided by technology, and enriched by the depth of understanding it fosters. It is a journey that transcends the conventional to explore the true potential of fasting as a catalyst for health and longevity.

REEVALUATING YOUR PLAN: WHEN TO MAKE CHANGES

In the quiet introspection accompanying the pursuit of health through intermittent fasting, there comes a time for recalibration when the efficacy of one's regimen demands scrutiny. The landscape of our bodies is one of constant flux, a terrain shaped by the interplay of biology, environment, and lifestyle. Within this dynamic framework, recognizing signs indicating the necessity for adjustment in one's fasting schedule becomes an act of attunement, a realignment with the evolving needs of the self. These subtle yet significant signs range from the stagnation of desired outcomes to shifts in vitality and alterations in overall health status. They whisper of the body's longing for change, a nudge toward adaptation in the face of new challenges or goals.

Adapting one's fasting regimen in response to these murmurs of need unfolds as a delicate operation, a fine-tuning of the mechanism by which we seek equilibrium. This process, far from merely altering timelines, is a re-engagement with the principles that underlie fasting, a recommitment to the dialogue between body and practice. Strategies for this adaptation encompass a spectrum of modifications, from restructuring fasting durations to exploring alternate fasting protocols. The objective remains constant: to invigorate the fasting experience and to rekindle the metabolic and cellular responses that initially marked the journey toward rejuvenation and health.

Incorporating feedback into the recalibration process emerges as a foundational element, a pillar upon which the edifice of a successful fasting regimen rests. This feedback, drawn from the wellspring of the body's reactions, health metrics tracked over time, and insights offered by medical advisors, forms a mosaic of data points. Each piece's unique implications contribute to a holistic understanding of the fasting journey's impact. Within this feedback, clues lie hidden—indicators of the body's responsiveness to fasting, its adaptability, and its needs. The integration of this feedback, a synthesis of internal and external insights, guides the fine-tuning of the fasting regimen, ensuring that the practice remains responsive to the individual's evolving landscape.

Cultivating a mindset oriented toward continuous improvement and experimentation defines the ethos of the intermittent fasting journey. This perspective, one of openness to the possibilities inherent in adjustment and adaptation, fosters a dynamic relationship with fasting. It encourages an exploratory approach to the practice, a willingness to test the boundaries of one's regimen to pursue optimal health and vitality. This mindset does not perceive modification as an admission of failure but as an affirmation of growth, a recognition that in the fluidity of life, our practices must remain fluid and adaptable to the currents of change.

In the quiet culmination of this chapter, the threads of reevaluation gather, weaving a narrative that speaks to the heart of the fasting journey. This narrative, enriched by the awareness of signs signaling the need for change, the strategies for adaptation, the integration of feedback, and the embrace of continuous improvement, frames fasting not as a static regimen but as a living practice. It underscores the importance of remaining attuned to the body's needs, listening to the whispers of change, and responding with intention and care. As we transition from this exploration of recalibration and adaptation, we carry forward the understanding that in the realm of health, as in life, transformation is not just a possibility but a promise, a horizon ever-expanding, inviting us to venture further into exploring our potential.

LOOKING AHEAD: SUSTAINING SUCCESS THROUGH ADAPTATION

A tapestry is only as enduring as the threads that bind it, woven with care to withstand the passage of time. Similarly, the fabric of our well-being, particularly as women over fifty, is crafted from the threads of knowledge, adaptation, and foresight. It is a fabric constantly under the loom, responsive to the shifting patterns of research, personal health, and the broader landscape of nutritional science. Within this framework, intermittent fasting is not static. Still, it evolves, a living testament to the dynamism of health and the pursuit of longevity.

THE FUTURE OF INTERMITTENT FASTING FOR WOMEN OVER 50

Emerging Research

The realm of intermittent fasting is vibrant with ongoing research, its potential unveiled through studies that cast light on long-term benefits yet to be fully understood. Imagine standing at the edge of a vast forest, the path ahead shrouded in mist. Each step reveals a new layer of the landscape, previously hidden from view. In this analogy, the forest is the burgeoning field of fasting research, and each step represents the advances in our understanding. Recent studies illuminate how fasting influences metabolism, cognitive function, and cellular repair mechanisms. These insights offer glimpses into uncharted territories of knowledge, promising avenues for enhancing health and extending vitality into later life.

Personalizing Fasting over Time

The imperative of tailoring fasting strategies to individual needs underscores the recognition that our bodies are landscapes of change. Like a gardener who adjusts to the seasons, introducing new crops and retiring others based on the rhythm of the year, practitioners of intermittent fasting must also remain attuned to the evolving needs of their bodies. This personalization necessitates a vigilant awareness of how one's health objectives shift with time, requiring adjustments to fasting schedules, dietary choices, and lifestyle factors to ensure that the practice continues to serve its intended purpose: fostering well-being and resilience.

The Evolving Landscape of Nutrition and Aging

Much like a river, nutritional science is ever-flowing, reshaped by the currents of new research and the sediment of accumulated knowledge. This fluid landscape influences the practice of intermittent fasting, particularly about aging. As we gain deeper insights into how nutritional needs transform with age, fasting protocols must adapt, reflecting the latest understanding of how best to support metabolic health, cognitive function, and cellular integrity. It is a dance of sorts, a responsive step to the melody of evolving science, ensuring that fasting practices remain aligned with the principles of optimal aging.

Anticipating Changes

Staying informed and adaptable in the face of emerging research is akin to a sailor navigating by the stars, ready to adjust the sails with the shifting winds. This readiness to adapt ensures that one's fasting practice remains at the forefront of health optimization, responsive to new discoveries and shifts in the scientific consensus. It involves a proactive engagement with the latest findings, a willingness to revise one's approach in light of new evidence, and a commitment to an ongoing dialogue with healthcare professionals. This approach not only maximizes the benefits of fasting but also safeguards against potential pitfalls, ensuring that the practice continues to be a pillar of health and vitality.

Visual Element: Interactive Timeline of Fasting Research

An interactive timeline detailing pivotal studies in intermittent fasting offers a visual journey through the research landscape. This timeline, accessible with the swipe of a finger, not only highlights key findings and their implications for women over fifty but also underscores the evolving nature of our understanding. It serves as both a resource and a reminder of the dynamic interplay between science and practice, encouraging readers to stay engaged with the unfolding story of intermittent fasting.

In the fabric of our well-being, intermittent fasting emerges as a thread woven with intention, responsive to the shifting patterns of research, personal health, and the evolving landscape of nutritional science. This adaptability, grounded in the pursuit of knowledge and the anticipation of change, ensures that intermittent fasting remains a vibrant and compelling component of health and longevity. As we navigate the complexities of this practice, the principles of personalization, responsiveness to research, and foresight guide us, crafting a tapestry of well-being that endures.

LIFELONG LEARNING: STAYING INFORMED ABOUT HEALTH TRENDS

Critical Evaluation of Information

In a landscape where the winds of health trends shift with relentless frequency, discerning the substance from the ephemeral becomes a skill of paramount importance. One must approach this task with the precision of an artisan, sifting through the trash of fleeting fads to uncover the grains of enduring wisdom. Strategies for this discernment necessitate a cultivated skepticism toward claims that seem too good to be true, favoring instead a reliance on the bedrock of peer-reviewed research and the medical community's consensus. It involves examining not just the results but also the methodology and looking behind the curtain to understand how conclusions were drawn. This critical evaluation serves as a beacon, guiding through the fog of sensationalism and marketing that too often obscures the truth.

Resources for Continuous Learning

To navigate the vast ocean of health information, one requires a compass—reputable resources that offer data and context, framing new findings within the broader narrative of health science. Esteemed publications such as the *New England Journal of Medicine* or *The Lancet* stand as lighthouses, illuminating the landscape with rigorous research and analysis. Websites like PubMed and the

National Institutes of Health offer portals to a world of studies and findings where the curious can delve deep into the specifics of intermittent fasting, nutrition, and the science of aging. For those seeking guidance distilled through the lens of practical application, organizations such as the Academy of Nutrition and Dietetics provide a bridge between the scientific community and the lay public, translating complex research into actionable advice.

Community Engagement

The journey through the evolving landscape of health trends should be undertaken in collaboration with others. Instead, it thrives on exchanging ideas, sharing experiences, and the collective pursuit of understanding. Engaging with virtual and physical communities creates a tapestry of support and learning, enriching the individual quest with the wisdom of many. Online forums dedicated to intermittent fasting and women's health burgeon with the stories of countless others navigating similar paths, offering insights, advice, and camaraderie. Local health seminars and workshops provide a space for connection and learning, where the abstract becomes tangible, and concepts are brought to life through discussion and demonstration. This engagement fosters a culture of shared knowledge, where learning is a communal act, and every question asked illuminates the path for others.

The Role of Professional Guidance

In the quest for health, the guidance of professionals serves as a keystone, anchoring the pursuit of well-being in a foundation of expertise and personalized care. Nutritionists, dietitians, and healthcare providers offer not just advice but partnership, collaborating with individuals to tailor fasting practices and dietary choices to the unique contours of their health landscape. While informed by the latest trends and research, this professional guidance is filtered through the lens of individual needs, creating a personalized roadmap that navigates the complexities of health optimization. Regular consultations ensure that this roadmap remains responsive to changing health indicators, new research findings, and the evolving goals of the individual. It is a dynamic process where professional expertise and personal insight converge to craft an informed and adaptable health strategy.

In this continuous journey of learning, the critical evaluation of information, the exploration of reputable resources, the engagement with communities, and the partnership with healthcare professionals create a multifaceted approach to staying informed about health trends. This approach, rooted in discernment, curiosity, and collaboration, ensures not just the acquisition of knowledge but the cultivation of wisdom, which guides the practice of intermittent fasting and the broader quest for vitality and well-being.

INTEGRATING NEW HABITS FOR LASTING CHANGE

Beyond Fasting

The act of weaving new habits into the fabric of daily life demands a finesse that transcends mere intention. It calls for a nuanced approach, where integrating practices such as mindfulness, routine physical exertion, and robust social interaction complements the discipline of intermittent fasting. This amalgamation of habits forms a synergy, each element enhancing the efficacy and enriching the experience of the others. Mindfulness, with its roots deep in the practice of present awareness, offers a foundation of calm and centeredness, vital for navigating the moments of challenge inherent in fasting. Routine physical exertion, whether it manifests through brisk walks in nature or structured sessions of yoga, fortifies the body, leveraging the physiological benefits fasting initiates. Robust social interaction—the threads that bind the human experience—provides a network of support and engagement vital for sustaining motivation and enriching the journey toward wellness.

Habit Stacking

The concept of habit stacking emerges as a potent tool in cultivating new routines, a methodical approach to layering practices that fosters adherence and amplifies benefits. For a moment, picture the deliberate construction of a stone cairn, each rock placed with care atop the last, creating a stable and symbolic structure. In habit stacking, each new habit becomes a stone, added to the foundation of existing routines, enhancing the overall structure of one's daily life. Drinking a glass of water upon waking, a simple yet effective habit can serve as a cue for a brief meditation session, which could precede a period of writing or reflection. This sequential chaining of habits creates a rhythm. This predictable pattern eases the incorporation of new behaviors into the established fabric of daily routines.

Overcoming Setbacks

The path to lasting change is seldom linear, marked by undulations and the occasional setback. These moments, while disheartening, offer invaluable opportunities for growth and recalibration. The key to navigating these challenges lies not in avoiding obstacles but in developing strategies for resilience. When faced with setbacks, a reflective pause to assess the precipitating factors provides clarity, allowing for a strategic response rather than a reactive retreat. Adjusting one's approach to fasting by modifying the fasting window or incorporating more gradual dietary changes reinvigorates stalled progress. Moreover, cultivating a mindset that views setbacks as temporary and informative rather than definitive can transform these obstacles into stepping stones, each a lesson on the journey toward lasting wellness.

Celebrating Progress

In pursuing health and vitality, the milestones achieved along the way deserve recognition and celebrations of progress that bolster spirit and resolve. These moments of acknowledgment serve as reminders of the journey's worth and the accumulated benefits of discipline and perseverance. Small victories, whether the successful integration of a new habit or a notable improvement in well-being, merit celebration. Creating rituals around these celebrations, perhaps a quiet evening of reflection or a shared meal with loved ones, imbues the journey with joy and a sense of accomplishment. In these celebrations, the essence of progress is distilled, a testament to the human capacity for growth and transformation.

In the intricate dance of habit formation and change, the integration of complementary practices, the strategic layering of routines, the resilience in the face of challenges, and the celebration of milestones weave together to form a tapestry of sustained transformation. This tapestry, rich with patterns of discipline, adaptability, and joy, frames the journey toward lasting wellness not as a series of isolated acts but as a cohesive narrative of growth and fulfillment.

THE ROLE OF MEDICAL SUPERVISION IN YOUR FASTING JOURNEY

In the intricate dance of health maintenance, the need for medical oversight emerges as a guiding light, illuminating the path for those navigating the waters of intermittent fasting, particularly for individuals whose health landscapes are marked by the contours of pre-existing conditions or the complexities of ongoing medication regimens. This oversight, far from a mere formality, stands as a beacon of safety and efficacy, ensuring that the practice of fasting is tailored to the unique physiological narratives of each individual.

The fabric of our well-being, woven from the threads of biology, habit, and aspiration, requires a keen eye for detail, an eye that healthcare professionals possess. Their expertise, honed through years of study and practice, offers a lens through which the nuances of fasting can be examined, understood, and optimized. Through this lens, the practice of intermittent fasting transcends the realm of general wellness to become a precision tool, shaped and refined to fit each person's individual needs and health objectives.

In collaborative health management, the partnership between individuals and their healthcare providers unfolds as a dynamic symphony, each participant bringing unique expertise. Here, armed with personal insights into their body's responses and health aspirations, the individual engages in an open dialogue with healthcare professionals. Together, they craft a fasting regimen that respects the individual's health background and current medication and aligns with their long-term wellness goals. This collaborative approach, characterized by mutual respect and shared decision-making, ensures that fasting becomes a harmonious element of a comprehensive health strategy rather than a discordant note.

Navigating health changes, an inevitable aspect of any wellness endeavor, demands a navigator skilled in reading the signs and adjusting the course. Healthcare providers, with their deep understanding of the body's signals and the potential implications of fasting, serve as invaluable guides in this journey. They offer insights into how fasting might interact with existing health conditions, providing adjustments to fasting schedules or dietary recommendations to mitigate risks and enhance benefits. Moreover, they can identify early signs of adverse reactions or unexpected benefits, allowing for timely interventions to ensure the fasting journey remains safe and fruitful. It is a journey of constant learning and adaptation, where the destination is not a static point but a state of optimized health and well-being.

Accessing professional resources becomes a critical step in securing the foundation for a safe and effective fasting practice. This access opens doors to a wealth of knowledge and expertise, from dietitians specialized in fasting protocols to endocrinologists with insights into hormonal balance and metabolism. Consultations with pharmacologists or primary care physicians become crucial for those taking medication. This ensures that fasting schedules are harmonized with medication regimens to prevent interactions or compromised efficacy. Furthermore, organizations such as the American Nutrition Association offer a repository of resources, from the latest research on fasting and metabolism to directories of healthcare professionals well-versed in the nuances of intermittent fasting. Seeking medical advice, particularly at the inception of a fasting journey or upon encountering health changes, stands as a pillar of responsible practice. This step safeguards health while maximizing the transformative potential of fasting.

In the vast landscape of intermittent fasting, where each individual's path is as unique as their fingerprints, the role of medical supervision cannot be overstated. It is a partnership that respects the complexity of the human body, recognizes the individuality of health journeys, and strives for optimization through personalization. This approach ensures that fasting, as a tool for health and vitality, is wielded with precision and care, guided by the expertise of professionals and the personal insights of each individual. It is through this collaborative endeavor that the true potential of intermittent fasting can be realized, offering a pathway to wellness that is both safe and profoundly effective.

EXPANDING YOUR HEALTH NETWORK: FINDING LIKE-MINDED COMMUNITIES

In the vast expanse of our quest for well-being, the solace found in the company of peers who share our aspirations can be a beacon during times of uncertainty and a celebration in moments of triumph. The value of community support, particularly for those navigating the complexities of intermittent fasting, cannot be overstated. Within these gatherings of minds and spirits, the solitary endeavor transforms into a shared pilgrimage toward health.

Benefits of Community Support

The tapestry of human interaction is rich with the threads of individual journeys, each woven into a larger narrative of collective experience. Reaching out and connecting with others who are also exploring the nuances of intermittent fasting brings forth many benefits. It is akin to finding oneself in a foreign land and discovering a fellow traveler who speaks your language. Suddenly, the journey feels less daunting, the path less treacherous. The exchange of knowledge, the sharing of hurdles overcome, and the collective brainstorming of strategies to navigate fasting's challenges foster a sense of solidarity. This camaraderie bolsters confidence, diminishes isolation, and imbues the fasting experience with a shared purpose.

Online Forums and Social Media

The digital age offers a labyrinth of pathways to connect with individuals across the globe, each seeking or offering wisdom on the art of intermittent fasting. Navigating this labyrinth requires discernment, for while it holds the promise of invaluable connections, it is also fraught with misinformation. Online forums dedicated to health, wellness, and specifically intermittent fasting serve as fertile ground for cultivating relationships with similar goals. Platforms such as Reddit and specialized fasting forums present opportunities to engage in discussions, pose questions, and offer insights from personal experience. Likewise, social media groups on platforms like Facebook and Instagram offer a wealth of shared knowledge and the visual inspiration of transformation stories. Engaging in these digital communities requires an openness to learn and share, coupled with a critical eye for the credibility of shared information. In these spaces, one can find solace and inspiration—a comforting reminder that others are navigating similar paths.

Local Groups and Events

While the digital realm offers broad connectivity, the power of in-person interaction remains unmatched. The tactile experience of meeting others embarking on or traversing the path of intermittent fasting enriches the journey in ways that digital engagement cannot replicate. Local health and wellness events, community seminars on nutrition and fasting, and even informal meet-up groups provide arenas for such connections. These gatherings allow for the exchange of ideas and experiences in a manner that nurtures trust and understanding. Sharing a space and engaging in a face-to-face conversation fosters a unique bond among participants. Within these local communities, the theoretical aspects of fasting practices can be discussed against the backdrop of real-world applications, where the abstract becomes tangible through shared meals or group fasting challenges.

Creating Your Own Community

When existing communities are sparse or misaligned with one's personal ethos, the initiative to forge a new collective presents itself as a bold but rewarding endeavor; creating a new community, be it virtual or physical, begins with articulating a vision—a clear, inviting depiction of the purpose and ethos of the gathering. This vision serves as a beacon, attracting individuals who resonate with the proposed ideals. Leveraging social media platforms, local community bulletin boards, or even word of mouth, one can extend an invitation to like-minded individuals seeking camaraderie on their fasting journey. The foundation of such a community rests on principles of mutual respect, openness to diverse experiences, and a shared commitment to support and uplift each other. Organizing regular meetings, whether online or in person, setting up group fasting challenges, and sharing resources and success stories can animate the community with a dynamic energy. It transforms the group from a mere assembly of individuals into a vibrant collective, enriched by the diversity of its members and united by a common quest for health and well-being.

In the vast expanse of our quest for well-being, finding and engaging with communities of like-minded individuals offers a tapestry of benefits—knowledge shared, support given and received, and the profound realization that one is not alone. Whether through digital forums, social media platforms, local groups, or the creation of new collectives, the value of community in the journey of intermittent fasting is immeasurable. Within these communities' embrace, the fasting journey transcends the individual, becoming a shared pilgrimage toward health and vitality.

CELEBRATING YOUR JOURNEY: REFLECTING ON HOW FAR YOU'VE COME

In the quiet spaces of introspection, the act of reflection unfurls as a delicate tapestry, each thread a testament to the growth, the hurdles surmounted, and the wisdom distilled from the practice of intermittent fasting. This reflective practice, far from a mere dalliance with memory, serves as a crucible for personal transformation, a mirror reflecting the intricate patterns of change woven through the fabric of our experiences. Acknowledging the milestones achieved, the lessons learned, and the resilience forged in the face of adversity, this act of reflection not only honors the distance traversed but also illuminates the path forward, casting light on the contours of future aspirations.

The sharing of one's narrative, the intimate tales of fasting's impact on body, mind, and spirit, resonates with the power of authenticity, a beacon for those navigating their own health odysseys. In the vulnerability of these shared stories, inspiration finds fertile ground, motivating both the storyteller and the listener to persist in their quests for well-being. These narratives, rich with the nuances of personal challenge and triumph, ripple through the fabric of our communities, a testament to the transformative potential of intermittent fasting. They serve not merely as accounts of personal achievement but as invitations to others to explore the possibilities inherent in their own lives.

The influence of these shared journeys extends beyond the individual, casting ripples across the pond of our collective experience. Friends, family, and the broader community, touched by the narrative of change, may find themselves inspired to adopt healthier behaviors, to explore the benefits of intermittent fasting, or to support their loved ones in their health endeavors. This ripple effect, subtle yet profound, underscores the interconnectedness of our health journeys, revealing how personal transformation can inspire communal shifts toward wellness. It is a reminder that our actions, our choices, and our stories hold the potential to influence the health landscape of our communities, seeding change that transcends the boundaries of individual experience.

Looking forward, the horizon of health and well-being stretches vast and inviting, a realm of possibilities awaiting exploration. The practice of intermittent fasting, enriched by the lessons of reflection, the inspiration drawn from shared narratives, and the communal shifts catalyzed by our journeys, stands as a beacon guiding us toward a future bright with the promise of vitality. This forward gaze, tempered by the wisdom of past experiences and buoyed by the support of our communities, infuses our ongoing quest for health with optimism and a sense of boundless potential. Within this landscape of possibility, we continue to weave the tapestry of our well-being, each thread a testament to the enduring power of transformation and the unyielding pursuit of vitality.

In the quiet afterglow of reflection, we stand at the threshold of continued exploration, our journeys marked by the milestones celebrated, the stories shared, and the communal impact of our health endeavors. This narrative, rich with the lessons of the past and the promise of the future, invites us to persist in our quest for well-being, ever mindful of the transformative power of our choices and the enduring influence of our shared journeys. As we close this chapter, let us carry forward the insights gleaned, the inspiration drawn, and the optimism kindled, stepping into the next phase of our exploration with confidence and a renewed commitment to health and vitality.

PAY IT FORWARD

I hope that as you end your journey through this book, you have already taken many steps to embark on the path of intermittent fasting. You have seen that each IF journey is unique and vast as it involves choosing the perfect window, foods, and exercise regimen that suits your lifestyle.

The good news is that taking the time to really think about what works for you is key if you wish to see long-term benefits such as weight loss, reduced stress levels, and stable hormone and blood sugar levels. And if you are inspired by what you've found within these pages, then I hope you can share your opinion with someone else.

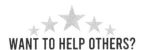

WANT TO HELP OTHERS?

Your story can inspire someone else to put their health in the spotlight, perhaps for the first time in their lives.

Thank you for your support. As stated so eloquently by the iconic actor, John Travolta, "You feel alive to the degree that you feel you can help others."

Scan the QR code to leave a review:

CONCLUSION

As we stand at the threshold of concluding our shared journey through *The Intermittent Fasting for Women Over 50 Revolution*, I find myself reflecting on the transformative power of intermittent fasting. It's been a profound exploration of how this approach can serve as a pivotal tool for managing weight, enhancing overall health, and gracefully navigating the challenges of menopause. The beauty of intermittent fasting lies in its flexibility. This customizable approach respects the unique needs, lifestyles, and rhythms of women over fifty.

I've emphasized the importance of holistic health integration, underscoring that true well-being extends far beyond dietary changes. By weaving intermittent fasting with balanced nutrition, regular physical activity, and practices that support mental and emotional well-being, we craft a comprehensive approach to sustainable health and aging with grace. This holistic tapestry, adorned with the threads of your individual needs and aspirations, is the foundation for lasting transformation.

Throughout our journey, we've revisited the significance of community and support. Remember, the power of connecting with a supportive network—online or in person—cannot be overstated. Sharing experiences, challenges, and successes with peers embarking on similar paths offers a motivational boost and a profound sense of belonging.

We've also tackled and debunked common myths and concerns about intermittent fasting, providing evidence-based explanations and practical advice to navigate these issues confidently. From addressing hormonal impacts to fasting schedules, my goal has been to equip you with the knowledge to make informed decisions on your wellness journey.

The inclusion of success stories from women over fifty who've thrived on intermittent fasting was intended to inspire and underscore the real-world applicability of this approach. These narratives serve as a beacon, illuminating the potential for profound personal transformation through intermittent fasting.

Now, as you stand on the cusp of starting—or perhaps continuing—your intermittent fasting journey, I encourage you to take that step confidently. Armed with the knowledge, strategies, and support outlined in this book, personalize your approach, be patient with yourself, and embrace this journey of discovery and transformation. Remember, each step is toward a healthier, more vibrant you.

Please view your intermittent fasting journey as an ongoing process of learning and adaptation. Stay curious, stay informed about the latest research, and remain open to adjusting your approach as needed. Your path to wellness is uniquely yours; let it evolve and flourish as you do.

In closing, I extend my deepest gratitude to you for joining me on this journey. Your commitment to exploring and embracing inter-mittent fasting as a pathway to health and vitality is both commendable and inspiring. Remember, you are not alone on this journey. The changes you are making today are investments in your future self—investments that I believe will yield incredible dividends in terms of health, vitality, and overall well-being.

Here's to you, your health, and the wonderful journey ahead. May it be filled with discovery, growth, and joy. Remember, the best is yet to come.

With gratitude and encouragement,

   - Eva Greenwell

BIBLIOGRAPHY

AMC Team. 2023. "How To Balance Your Hormones and Health With Yoga and Pilates During Menopause." *Australian Menopause Centre*. December 13. https://www.menopausecentre.com.au/information-centre/articles/how-to-balance-your-hormones-and-health-with-yoga-and-pilates-during/.

Bates, Autumn. 2022. "Intermittent Fasting Over 50: 5 Tips For Success." *AutumnElleNutrition*. April 6. https://www.autumnellenutrition.com/post/intermittent-fasting-over-50-5-tips-for-success.

BrainyQuote. "Help Others Quotes." Accessed March 30, 2024. https://www.brainyquote.com/topics/help-others-quotes

Brighten, Dr. Jolene. 2023. "Intermittent Fasting for Menopause: What You Need to Know to Before You Start." *Dr. Jolene Brighten*. December 29. https://drbrighten.com/intermittent-fasting-for-menopause/.

Brunt, Deborah. 2023. "The Best Anti-Inflammatory Diet for Menopause | Ōtepoti Integrative Health." *Otepoti Integrative*. March 31. https://www.otepotiintegrativehealth.co.nz/post/the-best-anti-inflammatory-diet-for-menopause.

Combs Dalton, Dr. Talita. 2022. "Intermittent Fasting Success Story: Fasting After Menopause." *Temper*. May 20. https://usetemper.com/learn/intermittent-fasting-success-story-fasting-after-menopause/.

Contributors, WebMD Editorial. 2024. "What to Know About Intermittent Fasting for Women After 50." *WebMD*. Accessed April 2. https://www.webmd.com/healthy-aging/what-to-know-about-intermittent-fasting-for-women-after-50.

Davidson, Katey. 2021. "The Definitive Guide to Healthy Eating in Your 50s and 60s." *Healthline*. September 20. https://www.healthline.com/nutrition/healthy-eating-50s-60s.

Davis, Jeanie Lerche. 2024. "Get-Fit Advice for Women Over 50." *WebMD*. Accessed April 2. https://www.webmd.com/women/women-over-50-fitness-tips.

Dr. T. Dalton Combs. 2022. "Intermittent Fasting Success Story: Fasting After Menopause." *Temper*. May 20. https://usetemper.com/learn/intermittent-fasting-success-story-fasting-after-menopause/.

Fletcher, Laura. 2022. "New Data on How Intermittent Fasting Affects Female Hormones." *UIC Today*. October 25. https://today.uic.edu/new-data-on-how-intermittent-fasting-affects-female-hormones/.

Gwinn, Alison. 2022. "8 Superfoods to Eat After 50." *AARP*. August 4. https://www.aarp.org/health/healthy-living/info-2021/superfoods-for-adult-health.html.

Holdaway, Megan, and Bessie O'Connor. 2024. "Nutrition Trends 2023." *Let's Eat Healthy*. Accessed April 2. https://www.healthyeating.org/nutrition-topics/nutrition-science/nutrition-trends/nutrition-trends-2023.

Isenmann, Eduard, Dominik Kaluza, Tim Havers, Ana Elbeshausen, Stephan Geisler, Katharina Hofmann, Ulrich Flenker, Patrick Diel, and Simon Gavanda. 2023. "Resistance Training Alters Body Composition in Middle-Aged Women Depending on Menopause - A 20-Week Control Trial." *BMC Women's Health* 23 (October): 526. doi:10.1186/s12905-023-02671-y.

Kashtanova, Daria A., Anastasiia N. Taraskina, Veronika V. Erema, Anna A. Akopyan, Mikhail V. Ivanov, Irina D. Strazhesko, Alexandra I. Akinshina, et al. 2022. "Analyzing Successful Aging and Longevity: Risk Factors and Health Promoters in 2020 Older Adults." *International Journal of Environmental Research and Public Health* 19 (13): 8178. doi:10.3390/ijerph19138178.

Markley, Lisa. 2023. "Habit Stacking: Build New Healthy Habits That Stick." *AdventHealth*. December 18. https://www.adventhealth.com/adventhealth-whole-health-institute/blog/habit-stacking-build-new-healthy-habits-stick.

McStay, Mara, Kelsey Gabel, Sofia Cienfuegos, Mark Ezpeleta, Shuhao Lin, and Krista A. Varady. 2021. "Intermittent Fasting and Sleep: A Review of Human Trials." *Nutrients* 13 (10): 3489. doi:10.3390/nu13103489.

Newcomb, Beth. 2024. "Fasting-Like Diet Lowers Risk Factors for Disease, Reduces Biological Age in Humans." *USC Leonard Davis School of Gerontology*. February 20. https://gero.usc.edu/2024/02/20/fasting-mimicking-diet-biological-age/.

Nguyen, Thao Thi Phuong, Hai Thanh Phan, Thuc Minh Thi Vu, Phuc Quang Tran, Hieu Trung Do, Linh Gia Vu, Linh Phuong Doan, et al. 2022. "Physical Activity and Social Support Are Associated with Quality of Life in Middle-Aged Women." *PLoS ONE* 17 (5): e0268135. doi:10.1371/journal.pone.0268135.

PhD, Dr T. Dalton Combs. 2022. "Intermittent Fasting Success Story: Fasting After Menopause." *Temper*. May 20. https://usetemper.com/learn/intermittent-fasting-success-story-fasting-after-menopause/.

Renae, Melissa. 2023. "Intermittent Fasting for Women Over 50 | A Guide by Simple." *Simple.Life Blog*. June 28. https://simple.life/blog/intermittent-fasting-for-women-over-50/.

Ruscio, Dr. Michael. 2022. "What to Know About Intermittent Fasting for Women Over 50." *Dr. Ruscio*. December 2. https://drruscio.com/fasting-for-women-over-50/.

Stella. 2022. "7-DAY INTERMITTENT FASTING MEAL PLAN (16/8 SCHEDULE)." *Beauty Bites*. January 3. https://www.beautybites.org/intermittent-fasting-meal-plan/.

Tabibzadeh, Siamak. 2023. "Role of Autophagy in Aging: The Good, the Bad, and the Ugly." *Aging Cell* 22 (1): e13753. doi:10.1111/acel.13753.

Tatiana. 2022. "6 Natural Ways to Balance Estrogen and Progesterone." *CT Hormone Therapy.* July 11. https://cthormonetherapy.com/6-natural-ways-to-balance-estrogen-and-progesterone/.

"The Nutrition Source." 2020. *Harvard School of Public Health.* September 14. https://www.hsph.harvard.edu/nutritionsource/mindful-eating/.

Top Right. "20 Transformational Quotes on Change Management." September 2, 2022. TopRight. https://toprightpartners.com/insights/20-transformational-quotes-on-change-management

University of Illinois Chicago. 2022. "How Intermittent Fasting Affects Female Hormones." *ScienceDaily.* October 25. https://www.sciencedaily.com/releases/2022/10/221025150257.htm.

Vetter, Christina. 2023. "Can Intermittent Fasting Improve Your Gut Health?" *Zoe.* August 2. https://zoe.com/learn/intermittent-fasting-gut-health.

Wong, Carmen, Benjamin Hon-Kei Yip, Ting Gao, Kitty Yu Yuk Lam, Doris Mei Sum Woo, Annie Lai King Yip, Chloe Yu Chin, et al. 2018. "Mindfulness-Based Stress Reduction (MBSR) or Psychoeducation for the Reduction of Menopausal Symptoms: A Randomized, Controlled Clinical Trial." *Scientific Reports* 8 (April): 6609. doi:10.1038/s41598-018-24945-4.

Yeager, Selene. 2022. "4 Reasons Why Menopausal Women Should Lift Heavy Sh*t." *Feisty Menopause.* March 23. https://www.feistymenopause.com/blog/liftheavyweights.

Yuan, Xiaojie, Jiping Wang, Shuo Yang, Mei Gao, Lingxia Cao, Xumei Li, Dongxu Hong, Suyan Tian, and Chenglin Sun. 2022. "Effect of Intermittent Fasting Diet on Glucose and Lipid Metabolism and Insulin Resistance in Patients with Impaired Glucose and Lipid Metabolism: A Systematic Review and Meta-Analysis." *International Journal of Endocrinology* 2022 (March): 6999907. doi:10.1155/2022/6999907.